LIST OF CONTRIBUTORS

£2.00

Dr J Dulay FRCP
Consultant Physician
Southampton University Hospital NHS Trust
Southampton

Dr CA Eynon FRCP
Director of Neurosciences Intensive Care
Wessex Neurological Centre
Southampton General Hospital
Southampton

Dr SE Fairbain MRCP(UK)
Specialist Respiratory Registrar
Llandough Hospital
South Wales

Dr L Keating MSc MRCP(UK)
Specialist Registrar in Emergency Medicine and Intensive Care
Milton Keynes General Hospital
Milton Keynes

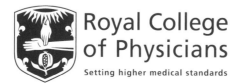
Royal College
of Physicians
Setting higher medical standards

Published by:
Royal College of Physicians of London
11 St. Andrews Place
Regent's Park
London NW1 4LE
United Kingdom

Set and printed by Graphicraft Limited, Hong Kong

First edition published 2001
Reprinted 2004
Second edition published 2008

ISBN: 978-1-86016-267-1 (this book)
ISBN: 978-1-86016-260-2 (set)

Distribution Information:
Jerwood Medical Education Resource Centre
Royal College of Physicians of London
11 St. Andrews Place
Regent's Park
London NW1 4LE
United Kingdom
Tel: +44 (0)207 935 1174 ext 422/490
Fax: +44 (0)207 486 6653
Email: merc@rcplondon.ac.uk
Web: http://www.rcplondon.ac.uk/

CONTENTS

FOREWORD

Since its initial publication in 2001, *Medical Masterclass* has been regarded as a key learning and teaching resource for physicians around the world. The resource was produced in part to meet the vision of the Royal College of Physicians: *'Doctors of the highest quality, serving patients well'*. This vision continues and, along with advances in clinical practice and changes in the format of the MRCP(UK) exam, has justified the publication of this second edition.

The MRCP(UK) is an international examination that seeks to advance the learning of and enhance the training process for physicians worldwide. On passing the exam physicians are recognised as having attained the required knowledge, skills and manner appropriate for training at a specialist level. However, passing the exam is a challenge. The pass rate at each sitting of the written papers is about 40%. Even the most prominent consultants have had to sit each part of the exam more than once in order to pass. With this challenge in mind, the College has produced *Medical Masterclass*, a comprehensive learning resource to help candidates with the preparation that is key to making the grade.

Medical Masterclass has been produced by the Education Department of the College. A work of this size represents a formidable amount of effort by the Editor-in-Chief – Dr John Firth – and his team of editors and authors. I would like to thank our colleagues for this wonderful educational product and wholeheartedly recommend it as an invaluable learning resource for all physicians preparing for their MRCP(UK) examination.

Professor Ian Gilmore MD PRCP
President of the Royal College of Physicians

PREFACE

The second edition of *Medical Masterclass* is produced and published by the Education Department of the Royal College of Physicians of London. It comprises 12 textbooks, a companion interactive website and two CD-ROMs. Its aim is to help doctors in their first few years of training to improve their medical knowledge and skills; and in particular to (a) learn how to deal with patients who are acutely ill, and (b) pass postgraduate examinations, such as the MRCP(UK) or European Diploma in Internal Medicine.

The 12 textbooks are divided as follows: two cover the scientific background to medicine, one is devoted to general clinical skills [including specific guidance on exam technique for PACES, the practical assessment of clinical examination skills that is the final part of the MRCP(UK) exam], one deals with acute medicine and the other eight cover the range of medical specialties.

The core material of each of the medical specialties is dealt with in seven sections:

- Case histories – you are presented with letters of referral commonly received in each specialty and led through the ways in which the patients' histories should be explored, and what should then follow in the way of investigation and/or treatment.

- Physical examination scenarios – these emphasise the logical analysis of physical signs and sensible clinical reasoning: 'having found this, what would you do?'

- Communication and ethical scenarios – what are the difficult issues that commonly arise in each specialty? What do you actually say to the 'frequently asked (but still very difficult) questions?'

- Acute presentations – what are the priorities if you are the doctor seeing the patient in the Emergency Department or the Medical Admissions Unit?

- Diseases and treatments – structured concise notes.

- Investigations and practical procedures – more short and to-the-point notes.

- Self assessment questions – in the form used in the MRCP(UK) Part 1 and Part 2 exams.

The companion website – which is continually updated – enables you to take mock MRCP(UK) Part 1 or Part 2 exams, or to be selective in the questions you tackle (if you want to do ten questions on cardiology, or any other specialty, you can do). For every question you complete you can see how your score compares with that of others who have logged onto the site and attempted it. The two CD-ROMs each contain 30 interactive cases requiring diagnosis and treatment.

I hope that you enjoy using *Medical Masterclass* to learn more about medicine, which – whatever is happening politically to primary care, hospitals and medical career structures – remains a wonderful occupation. It is sometimes intellectually and/or emotionally very challenging, and also sometimes extremely rewarding, particularly when reduced to the essential of a doctor trying to provide best care for a patient.

John Firth DM FRCP
Editor-in-Chief

ACKNOWLEDGEMENTS

Medical Masterclass has been produced by a team. The names of those who have written or edited material are clearly indicated elsewhere, but without the support of many other people it would not exist. Naming names is risky, but those worthy of particular note include: Sir Richard Thompson (College Treasurer) and Mrs Winnie Wade (Director of Education), who steered the project through committees that are traditionally described as labyrinthine, and which certainly seem so to me; and also Arthur Wadsworth (Project Co-ordinator) and Don Liu in the College Education Department office. Don is a veteran of the first edition of *Medical Masterclass*, and it would be fair to say that without his great efforts a second edition might not have seen the light of day.

John Firth DM FRCP
Editor-in-Chief

KEY FEATURES

We have created a range of icon boxes that sit among the text of the various *Medical Masterclass* modules. They are there to help you identify key information and to make learning easier and more enjoyable. Here is a brief explanation:

> Iron-deficiency anaemia with a change in bowel habit in a middle-aged or older patient means colonic malignancy until proved otherwise.

This icon is used to highlight points of particular importance.

> Dietary deficiency is very rarely, if ever, the sole cause of iron-deficiency anaemia.

This icon is used to indicate common or important drug interactions, pitfalls of practical procedures, or when to take symptoms or signs particularly seriously.

ACUTE MEDICINE

Authors:

J Dulay, CA Eynon, SE Fairbain and L Keating

Editor:

CA Eynon

Editor-in-Chief:

JD Firth

PACES STATIONS AND ACUTE SCENARIOS

1.1 Communication skills and ethics

1.1.1 Cardiac arrest

> **Scenario**
>
> **Role**: you are a junior doctor on the cardiac arrest team.
>
> A 75-year-old man, Mr Tony Foster, has suffered a cardiac arrest on the ward. He was admitted 3 days previously with an inferior myocardial infarction. Unfortunately resuscitation attempts have been futile.
>
> **Your task**: the nurses have asked you to speak to Mr Foster's wife and explain that her husband has died.

Key issues to explore

It is vital to find out what the wife knows already: she may have just arrived spontaneously without any warning of what has been going on; alternatively the nursing staff may have phoned to explain that her husband is very poorly and that she should come to the hospital immediately.

Key points to establish

- Get the setting right: ideally you need a quiet room adjacent to the ward where you are not going to be interrupted. Ensure that you have left your bleep (and mobile phone) with a colleague. Take one of the senior ward nurses as support (both for the family and yourself). The room should ideally have a supply of tissues and a telephone.

- Introductions: ensure you have introduced yourself and what you do; also introduce any nursing or other hospital staff who are with you.

- Ensure you have the correct family and know precisely who you are speaking to: many of us have had the misfortune to break news to a daughter thinking it was the patient's wife, or vice versa.

- Be explicit about what has happened: that the patient's heart stopped suddenly; that the cardiac arrest team was called; that attempts were made to resuscitate the patient; but that these were unsuccessful and that unfortunately Mr Foster has died.

- It is important to listen: give his wife time to understand and to ask questions.

Appropriate responses to likely questions

Wife: why has this happened?

Doctor: as a result of the heart attack, your husband's heart had become weaker. Just after a heart attack the heart is irritable and the normal pattern of the heartbeat can be disrupted, which can lead it to stop pumping blood properly to the brain and other organs.

Wife: what did you do?

Doctor: as soon as the team on the ward recognised that his heart had stopped, they called the cardiac arrest team. He was given oxygen and heart massage – pressing up and down on the chest to keep the blood moving in the body – and he was defibrillated which is a special electric shock to try to get the heart beating steadily again. He was also given various drugs to try to help, but I'm afraid that these didn't work. The damage to his heart was obviously too great.

Wife: would he have felt any pain?

Doctor: no: patients become unconscious very quickly as soon as this happens. During the resuscitation attempts he showed no signs of life and will not have felt any pain.

Wife: but on the television resuscitation is usually successful.

Doctor: yes, I know, but in real life the heartbeat only returns in about 30% of people who have a cardiac arrest in hospital, and only around half of those survive to reach hospital discharge. I agree that things go well on the television more often, but unfortunately the figures are much lower in real life.

Further comments

Which deaths require reporting to the coroner (procurator fiscal in Scotland)?

- Cause of death is unknown.

- Deceased was not seen by the certifying doctor either after death or within the 14 days before death.

- Death was violent, unnatural or suspicious.

- Death may be due to an accident (whenever that occurred).

- Death may be due to self-neglect or neglect by others.

- Death may be due to an industrial disease or related to the person's employment.

- Death may be due to an abortion.

- Death occurred during an operation or before recovery from the effects of anaesthetic.

- Suicide.

- Death occurred during or shortly after detention in police or prison custody.

Who should be notified following a cardiac arrest?

- The coroner may be required to be notified (see above).

- The patient's GP.

- The consultant responsible for the management of the patient should be notified as soon as possible.

Who fills in the death certificate?

- Part 1 should be completed by one of the medical team caring for the patient. It should include the date of death and details as to the presumed cause. It has sections detailing whether information is available (or may become available later) from a post-mortem and whether the coroner has been informed.

- Part 2 is completed by a medical practitioner with at least 5 years of experience. Following the Shipman enquiry, the person completing part 2 will contact not only the person completing part 1 but also one of the nursing staff or another medical practitioner involved in the case to ensure there were no suspicious circumstances.

1.1.2 Stroke

Scenario

Role: you are a junior medical doctor on-call for the wards.

An 80-year-old man, Mr Anand Patel, has been admitted to hospital with a dense left hemispheric stroke resulting in aphasia and a right hemiparesis. He has a background history of prostatic carcinoma, left ventricular failure, atrial fibrillation and chronic obstructive pulmonary disease. His Glasgow Coma Scale score has fallen to 7 (E2, M4, V1), which is presumed to be due to an extension of his stroke. The consultant has reviewed the patient and feels that intensive care unit (ICU) care is inappropriate and that the patient should not be resuscitated in the event of cardiopulmonary arrest.

Your task: you are asked to explain to the family what has happened and why it would be inappropriate to attempt resuscitation in the event of cardiopulmonary arrest.

Key issues to explore

What preparations should you make before speaking to the family?

- Obtain as much information as possible about the patient's comorbidities and functional level before his stroke: in PACES

scrutinise the scenario very carefully for details; in routine clinical practice look through the notes and speak to any staff present who may be able to give you useful information. This is essential, not only to inform appropriate decision-making, but also in discussing the issue with the family. They are much more likely to accept advice from a doctor who clearly knows the patient, Mr Patel, rather than one who seems to regard him as 'just another old man who's had a big stroke'.

- The scenario states that ICU care is not appropriate, but if that is so then what care is to be given? If the patient were to develop a chest infection, are you are going to try a course of antibiotics or is only comfort care indicated? These issues may be spelled out in a PACES scenario, but in routine clinical practice it is very important to establish and agree amongst the medical and nursing team exactly what treatments will and will not be given before embarking on discussions with a patient's relatives.

- What do the family know already and what are their expectations? They may have expected Mr Patel to make a full recovery with supportive care.

Key points to establish

- Get the setting right: ideally you need a quiet room adjacent to the ward where you are not going to be interrupted. Ensure that you have left your bleep (and mobile phone) with a colleague. Take one of the senior ward nurses as support (both for the family and yourself). The room should ideally have a supply of tissues and a telephone.

- Introductions: ensure you have introduced yourself and what you do; introduce any nursing or other hospital staff who are with you.

- Ensure you have the correct family and know precisely who you are speaking to.

- Be explicit about what has happened: the patient has had a severe stroke that has resulted in paralysis and loss of speech, and despite supportive measures his condition has deteriorated and he is now semi-conscious.

- Be explicit about your management plan: you are going to ensure that he is comfortable, with enough analgesia (if required) and fluids to ensure that he will not be distressed. The priority is to maintain his comfort and dignity.

- Be explicit about the limits of care that will be given: that increasing the level of care is felt to be futile, and that ventilation or cardiopulmonary resuscitation would not alter the outcome (families are often very relieved that their loved one will not be put through distressing 'treatments' for no effect).

- Listen: give the family time to understand and to ask questions.

Appropriate responses to likely questions

Relative: why has this happened?

Doctor: as a result of the stroke, he has very severe weakness of the right side of his body and he has lost his speech. After a stroke as big as this the brain sometimes becomes progressively more swollen, which makes things worse, and the patient becomes more deeply unconscious.

Relative: is he going to get better?

Doctor: I'm sorry to have to say this, but I don't think he is. He's had a very big stroke and things seem to be getting worse. I'd be delighted to be wrong, but I don't think he's going to recover. I'm afraid that I think he's going to die.

Relative: is he in any pain?

Doctor: no, I don't think he is. I think he is too deeply unconscious to be aware of what's happening or to be in any pain. Our priority is to make sure that he is comfortable, and if we thought he was in pain or was distressed, we would give him painkillers to prevent him from being in any pain or discomfort.

Relative: if he gets worse, are you just going to let him die?

Doctor: the most important thing is that we make sure that he's not in any pain or distress. You are right that sometimes doing cardiac massage – CPR – and putting people onto breathing machines can be helpful. However, doing this is only kind and sensible if you have a condition that you can reverse with treatment and in this case I'm afraid that the effects of the stroke are not going to be reversible. Ventilation and CPR would not have any effect on his underlying condition. We will ensure that he is comfortable and not in any pain.

1.1.3 Congestive cardiac failure

Scenario

Role: you are a junior doctor working as evening cover on a general medical ward.

Mr Harold Wilson is 89 years old. He had a stroke 5 years ago and is a diabetic on insulin. He lives at home with his son, but has been house-bound since his stroke. He was admitted 5 days ago with congestive cardiac failure. Medical therapy has been instituted, including oxygen, diuretics, fluids and vasodilators. There has been no response to treatment. He has become increasingly short of breath and is hypoxic despite oxygen. He has not passed urine for 4 hours. His Glasgow Coma Scale score is currently 8. He was reviewed by the consultant on the ward round who decided that he should be managed conservatively and not resuscitated in the event of cardiac arrest. His son was involved in the decision. It is now 9 p.m. and Mr Wilson's daughter has arrived: she feels that her father should be on the intensive care unit (ICU).

Your task: to explain to the daughter that transferring her father to the ICU would not be appropriate.

Key issues to explore

What does the daughter believe is likely to happen to her father? Why does she want him transferred to the ICU?

Key points to establish

- What does she know about her father's condition and his previous state of health? She does not live with him and may not be aware of these things.

- Explain what treatment has been given: he has been treated actively but has deteriorated despite this.

- Be explicit about the prognosis: her father is dying and there is no treatment that will prevent this. Futile treatments (such as resuscitation or transfer to ICU) will not be given.

- Explain the management plan: her father will be given treatments to alleviate his symptoms and to ensure that he is comfortable and dignified (some people may be worried that a 'Do not resuscitate' order means that no treatment will be given).

Appropriate responses to likely questions

Daughter: why isn't he on the intensive care unit?

Doctor: I'm sorry to have to tell you that your father is dying. He has been given treatment for his heart with oxygen, diuretics – drugs to get fluid out of the body – and other drugs to help the heart beat more strongly, but despite all of these the situation is deteriorating. Your father's heart, lungs, kidneys and brain are all failing. There is no treatment that will reverse this, on the ICU or anywhere else; nothing that will alter the final outcome.

Daughter: is there nothing more you can do for him?

Doctor: we can try to make his breathing easier for him, we can make sure that he is comfortable and dignified, and we will ensure that he is not in any pain.

Daughter: you are only saying this because that's what my brother thinks.

Doctor: no, that's not true. We have spoken about things with your brother, and he does agree with our plan for treatment. But decisions about treatment are made us, by the medical team, and not by your brother or anyone else. We have made what we think is the right plan.

Daughter: can I speak to someone more senior about this?

Doctor: yes, I can arrange that. The consultant saw your father earlier today on the ward round. She is aware of your father's condition, and the plan that I have outlined to you is the one that she made. However, she is not in the hospital at the moment. If you would like to speak to someone right away, then I can find out if the on-call registrar is available to answer any questions you may have that I cannot answer, or if one of the doctors on the ICU could speak to you, but I'm sure that they will tell you what I've already said. I'm very sorry. I'd like to be able to say something different, but your father is dying and we must make sure he's comfortable.

1.1.4 Lumbar back pain

Scenario

Role: you are a junior doctor on the medical assessment unit.

You have taken a history and examined a 40-year-old man, Mr Chris Pitman, who called 999 with severe lumbar back pain. He is usually fit and well, but has a 2-day history of pain radiating down his left leg. There are no red flags in the history or on examination. Examination confirms a diagnosis of mechanical back pain. You have prescribed appropriate analgesia. On review, his pain has settled and you want to discharge him to the care of his GP. He is insistent that he needs X-rays prior to discharge.

Your task: to explain to the patient that no further investigation is needed at this stage and that he can be discharged back to his GP for follow-up with referral to physiotherapy if required.

Key points to explore

What is the patient's main worry? Why does he want further investigation?

Key points to establish

- The history and examination have given reassuring results: the pain is not sinister; he does not have cancer of the spine (or any similar problem).

- Further tests are not indicated at this stage.

- There are simple strategies for coping with the pain.

- What to do if the pain fails to settle.

Appropriate responses to likely questions

Patient: can you guarantee this pain won't come back?

Doctor: no, I'm afraid that unfortunately I can't guarantee that. The prognosis for mechanical back pain is good, with 90% of sufferers recovering by 6 weeks, but recurrence is common.

Patient: how do you know I don't have anything seriously wrong with me without an X-ray?

Doctor: I'm afraid that an X-ray will not be helpful here. As I've said, I don't think that there is a sinister problem: I don't think that you have cancer of the spine or anything like that. But even if you did, then it's extremely unlikely that a simple X-ray would show anything. You'd need other special scans.

Patient: so shouldn't I have the special scans then?

Doctor: no, I don't think so. The chances of them showing anything would be extremely small and they are not without risks: some of these scans would expose you to radiation. However, if the pain continues beyond 6 weeks then the matter should be reconsidered. It is important that you arrange to see your GP when you get home, so that he or she can review your symptoms and see if anything further needs to be done at that time.

Patient: is there nothing you can do for me?

Doctor: yes, there is. I can give you some strong painkillers, some anti-inflammatories and some tablets to help muscle spasm. All of these can help and it is advisable for you to stay as active as possible. Even simple exercises can help. Your family doctor could organise a referral to a physiotherapist if things don't settle down quickly.

1.1.5 Community-acquired pneumonia

Scenario

Role: you are a junior doctor on call in the acute medical assessment unit.

Mr Chang, aged 35, has been referred by his GP with chest pain, malaise, lethargy and a productive cough. His symptoms have been present for 4 days. He is otherwise fit and well, and takes no regular medication. He is a smoker of 20 cigarettes per day. Investigations have shown that he has right lower lobe pneumonia, and his CURB-65 score is 0/5 (the British Thoracic Society guidelines scoring system, indicating non-severe pneumonia in this case). You feel that his illness could be managed at home, but he thinks he should be admitted for treatment.

Your task: to explain the nature of his illness and treatment plan, including discharge with continued treatment at home.

Key issues to explore

What are the patient's concerns regarding discharge? Are there any problems with regards to discharge and recuperation at home? Is there a support network available if he is discharged?

Key points to establish

- Explain the diagnosis and that the treatment plan is in line with current national recommendations.

- Explore issue of smoking cessation in light of the patient's current illness.

- Give details of who he should contact if he has any concerns, and suggest reattendance if any there are problems.

- Explain follow-up plans after discharge.

Appropriate responses to likely questions

Patient: would I not be better off staying in hospital?

Doctor: no, I don't think so. The investigations have shown us that you have an uncomplicated pneumonia, and we have started the appropriate antibiotics and expect that your symptoms will improve over the next few days. I'm pleased to say that you do not have any signs of severe pneumonia, and your treatment can be safely carried out at home.

Patient: you only want to send me home because there aren't any beds in the hospital.

Doctor: I can understand why you might say this, but it's not true. If we felt that you needed to be admitted for treatment, then we would do so.

Patient: are you going to blame my smoking?

Doctor: yes, I am, at least partly. People who don't smoke can get pneumonia, but smoking damages some of the mechanisms that clear infection from the lungs, so as a smoker you are more prone to respiratory illnesses. Smoking will also delay your recovery from such an illness, so it is important to consider stopping seriously. If you want to try to do this, I would suggest that you discuss matters with your GP or contact one of the relevant support groups.

Patient: what if my symptoms deteriorate and I don't get better?

Doctor: as I said, I don't expect your symptoms to deteriorate. However, if things do not improve or if there are any problems then you should contact your GP for advice. And if things got really bad, which I am not expecting, then you could come back up to the Emergency Department, although I think it very unlikely that this will be necessary.

Patient: if I go home, will I need any follow-up?

Doctor: yes, if all goes well it would be sensible for you to organise an appointment with your GP to get checked over in a few weeks' time. They will listen to your chest and organise a chest X-ray to check that everything has cleared up as expected.

1.1.6 Acute pneumothorax

Scenario

Role: you are a junior doctor on call in the acute medical assessment unit.

Mrs Diane Johnson, aged 36 years, is complaining of mild, right-sided chest pain. She is normally fit and well and is a lifelong non-smoker. On examination she is comfortable at rest and is not breathless. Her pulse rate is 85 bpm, her respiration rate 14/minute and her oxygen saturation is 98% (on air). On auscultation there are reduced breath sounds on the right. A CXR reveals a small right-sided pneumothorax. You are happy to discharge her with no further intervention, but with a recommendation to avoid strenuous exercise (also flying and diving) until review, which you have arranged in 2 weeks. She wants further treatment and feels she needs to be admitted. Her husband is also very concerned.

Your task: to explain to Mrs Johnson and her husband that no further intervention is required and that it is safe to discharge her.

Key issues to explore

What are their concerns regarding treatment and planned discharge? Is an appropriate environment and support network accessible on discharge?

Key points to establish

- Explain the diagnosis, and the reasons for observation versus further intervention.

- Give advice on activity limitation, ie flying, diving and strenuous exercise.

- Explain that in the unlikely event of deteriorating symptoms, she needs to reattend.

- Explain follow-up arrangements.

Appropriate responses to likely questions

Patient: why are you not going to treat me?

Doctor: there are treatments that could remove the small amount of the air that has leaked into your chest, but these involve putting needles or tubes through the chest wall and so they are not without risk. We use them only when patients have a bigger pneumothorax than yours – so large that it makes them breathless – or the lung is very collapsed on the chest X-ray. I'm pleased to say that you have only got a small pneumothorax on the chest X-ray and it's not making you breathless. Therefore, the best advice is to wait: in 80% of cases it will get better on its own.

Patient: what if I get more symptoms when I am at home?

Doctor: it is unlikely that you will, but if you get more breathless or if the pain gets worse, then you should come back to the hospital immediately.

Patient: if I go home, when will you see me again?

Doctor: we will arrange for you to be seen in outpatients in 2 weeks' time, with a repeat chest X-ray. If there are any concerns prior to this, contact us or your GP. As I've already said, if you have more breathlessness or chest pain you should reattend immediately.

Patient: what are the chances of this happening again?

Doctor: you are right in thinking that if you have had one pneumothorax then you are at greater risk of having another one than someone who has never had the problem at all. It's difficult to put a figure on this, but the chances of you having another pneumothorax are probably about 30–40%. But the fact that you do not smoke and are fit and well reduces your risk of recurrence.

Patient: we're planning to go on holiday to Spain in 4 months' time to celebrate our wedding anniversary. Is this OK?

Doctor: yes, it's important that you inform your travel insurance company – you should always do this if there's a significant change in your medical condition – but it should be all right for you to travel. The standard advice is that you should not fly for 6 weeks following complete resolution of a pneumothorax, and diving on holiday, which changes the air pressure in your lungs, is not recommended.

1.2 Acute scenarios

1.2.1 Cardiac arrest

Scenario

A 75-year-old man is found collapsed in bed on the ward. He was admitted 3 days previously with an inferior myocardial infarction. You are called as a member of the cardiac arrest team.

Introduction

Confirmation of cardiac arrest

Confirmation of cardiac arrest

- Shake the patient and ask loudly 'Are you OK? Can you hear me?'
- If there is no response, then shout for help.
- Open the airway: use the head-tilt, chin lift method (or if trauma is suspected, use the jaw thrust method).

- Check for signs of normal breathing and feel for the carotid pulse (<10 seconds).
- If the patient has no signs of life, is not breathing, has no pulse or if there is any doubt, send someone for help; if you are on your own, leave the victim and alert the resuscitation team/ambulance service. Start chest compressions, combining them with rescue breathing at a rate of 30:2.

⚠
- Checking the carotid pulse is an inaccurate method of confirming cardiac arrest: if in doubt commence cardiopulmonary resuscitation (CPR).
- Agonal breaths are common immediately following sudden cardiac arrest and should not delay commencement of CPR.

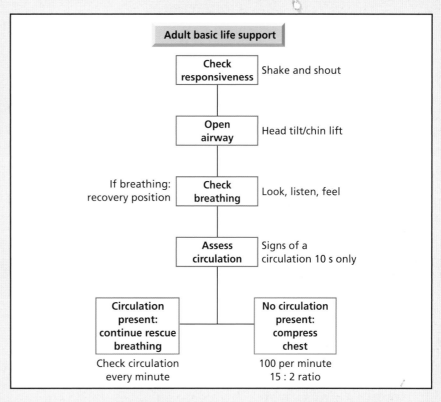

▲ **Fig. 1** European Resuscitation Council (ERC) guidelines for single-rescuer BLS.

Who should be resuscitated?

Cardiorespiratory arrest is common to all causes of death, but CPR should only be attempted if there is a potentially reversible cause for the arrest. An attempt should be made to resuscitate all patients unless a 'Do not resuscitate' (DNR) order has been written in the nursing and medical notes. In an acute situation decisions about CPR should be made by the most senior medical person present at the time, and discussed with the consultant in charge of the case at the earliest opportunity. If the clinical condition of a patient alters, then decisions about CPR and/or DNR orders should be reconsidered. It is good practice to discuss CPR decisions with both the patient and relatives if possible.

⚠
Many patients are concerned that a DNR order implies that nothing will be done, even to the extent of withholding analgesia and fluids in the event of their decline. They must be strongly reassured that this is not so.

Management

Basic life support

Basic life support (BLS) comprises initial assessment, maintenance of a patent airway, rescue breathing and closed-chest compressions (Fig. 1). The primary objective is to provide sufficient oxygenated blood to the brain and heart until definitive therapy can be applied and spontaneous circulation re-established. BLS is a holding method only, but it at least doubles the chances of survival if applied between the time of collapse and first defibrillation.

Cardiac output during CPR ranges from one-quarter to one-third of normal. Diastolic BP and consequently coronary perfusion pressure falls rapidly after the first few minutes of CPR.

Advanced life support

Advanced life support (ALS) consists of definitive airway management and the use of drugs and defibrillation to attempt to re-establish a spontaneous cardiac output (Fig. 2). Traditionally an endotracheal tube (a cuffed airway placed within the trachea to enable both oxygenation and ventilation) was used to provide a definitive airway. The ease of placement of the laryngeal mask airway means that it is now more widely used, although it can potentially result in a higher risk of aspiration.

Categories of cardiac arrest

Two major categories are recognised: (i) ventricular fibrillation or pulseless ventricular tachycardia (VF and VT, respectively) and (ii) non-VF/VT (previously subdivided into asystole and pulseless electrical activity).

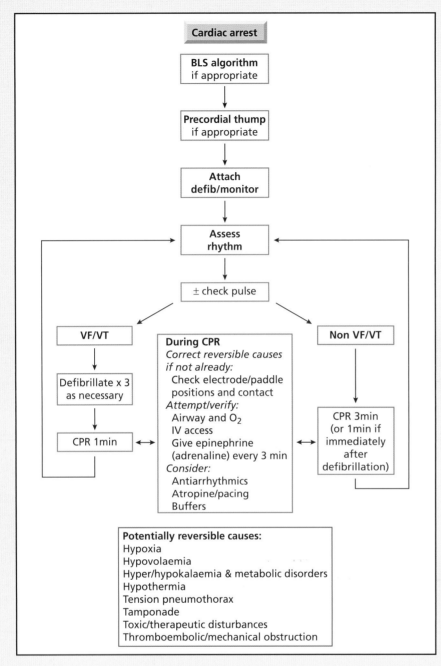

▲**Fig. 2** ERC guidelines for ALS.

Note the following.

- If a perfusing rhythm is present on reassessing the ECG on the monitor, try to palpate a pulse. Rhythm checks should be brief and pulse checks only performed if a perfusing rhythm is present.

- If an organised rhythm is present during a period of CPR, do not suspend the CPR unless the patient starts to show signs of life. If a perfusing rhythm has been restored, giving chest compressions does not increase the chances of VF recurring.

- If VF/VT persists after three shocks, give amiodarone 300 mg iv.

Treatment of non-VF/VT

- Recommence CPR.
- Check electrode/paddle positions and contact.
- Obtain and secure the patient's airway and administer high-flow oxygen.
- Obtain intravenous access.
- Administer 1 mg epinephrine (adrenaline) intravenously every 3–5 minutes.
- Assess for potentially reversible causes.
- Reassess rhythm and defibrillate as necessary.

Epinephrine (adrenaline) is the first-line vasopressor, although it has not been shown to improve survival. Vasopressin is an alternative, but its use is not widespread.

Potentially reversible causes of non-VF/VT

- Hypoxia: ensure 100% oxygen is being administered, preferably via an endotracheal tube or laryngeal mask airway.

- Hypovolaemia: administer a rapid fluid bolus of 500–1000 mL 0.9%

Treatment of VF/pulseless VT

- As soon as a defibrillator arrives, apply the paddles or self-adhesive pads to the chest.
- Give one shock (150–200 J biphasic or 360 J monophasic).
- Do not reassess the rhythm or check for a pulse.
- Resume CPR for 2 minutes, then reassess the ECG on the monitor.

- If VF is still present, give a second shock (150–200 J biphasic or 360 J monophasic).
- Resume CPR for 2 minutes, then reassess the ECG on the monitor.
- If VF is still present, give 1 mg epinephrine (adrenaline) intravenously and then a third shock (150–200 J biphasic or 360 J monophasic).
- Resume CPR for 2 minutes, then reassess the ECG on the monitor.

saline; palpate for an abdominal aortic aneurysm; and check for rectal bleeding.

- Hypokalaemia/hyperkalaemia and metabolic disorders: check the patient's clinical history (if available) for clues. If the patient has a known renal disease, presume hyperkalaemia is present and give 10 mL of 10% calcium chloride or calcium gluconate intravenously.

- Hypothermia: the patient is never dead until warm and dead.

- Tension pneumothorax: consider especially in patients with pre-existing lung disease or in those on a ventilator. Look for asymmetrical chest, deviated trachea and unilateral absence of breath sounds. Immediate needle decompression of the affected side is mandatory.

- Tamponade: diagnosis is difficult. There is nothing to lose by attempting pericardiocentesis.

- Toxins including drug overdose: check clinical history for clues.

- Pulmonary embolism: always consider as a potential primary diagnosis.

Further comments

Antiarrhythmics in the management of cardiac arrest

There is no clear evidence for the use of antiarrhythmics in cardiac arrest. Although atropine is of use for haemodynamically significant bradycardia, its use in asystole is based on limited data. In cases of VF, amiodarone administered following three initial shocks has been shown to improve the short-term survival of patients until hospital admission compared with placebo or lidocaine (lignocaine).

What role do buffers have in the management of cardiac arrest?

Adequate ventilation and tissue perfusion is the best way to treat the combined metabolic and respiratory acidosis seen in cardiac arrest. In specific cases of arrest associated with tricyclic antidepressant overdose, hyperkalaemia and pre-existing metabolic acidosis, giving sodium bicarbonate intravenously may be of benefit.

What role does pacing have in the management of cardiac arrest?

External pacing of asystole has shown no clinical benefit. Pacing may be of occasional use for the treatment of ventricular standstill.

Outcome following cardiac arrest

Return of spontaneous circulation (ROSC) occurs in about 30% of in-hospital cardiac arrests, but only around 15% of patients survive to hospital discharge. Only 2% of out-of-hospital arrests survive to hospital discharge. The survival rate for VF/VT is 10–15 times higher than for non-VF/VT. Survival from VF/VT correlates with the time taken before the first shock is applied, with an approximately 10% reduction in patient survival for each minute taken. Over 80% of patients resuscitated from VF/VT are done so with one of the first three shocks.

If you are successful in resuscitating the patient, what should be done?

- Transfer to an appropriate area for monitoring and treatment.

- Monitoring: ECG, Sao$_2$ and non-invasive BP.

- Treatment: high-flow oxygen.

- Debrief of the medical team and nursing staff involved (a nominated person should complete a cardiac arrest audit

form if it is standard hospital practice).

- Routine investigations: ECG, electrolytes, renal function, CXR and arterial blood gases.

- Other investigations: pursue reversible factors as dictated by clinical suspicion.

If the patient remains unconscious, transfer to the intensive care unit or neuro critical care unit (NCCU) is required if active management is to be pursued. Cerebral cooling may be considered: two randomised trials have shown improved outcome in unconscious adult patients with spontaneous circulation after out-of-hospital VF arrest who were cooled to 32–34°C. This is thought to suppress reperfusion injury. It is unclear whether cooling is beneficial for patients who remain unconscious after resuscitation from other rhythms.

When should an unsuccessful attempt at CPR be stopped?

If ROSC does not occur promptly, consideration must be given to termination of the attempt. Delays of more than 5 minutes before the start of BLS or more than 30 minutes to defibrillation are associated with a very poor prognosis. The presence of systemic sepsis, disseminated cancer and major organ failure are also predictors of very poor outcome. Age itself is not an independent predictor for the success of resuscitation, but comorbidities are more common and result in lower survival rates in the elderly. Hypothermia and the ingestion of some cerebral depressants (sedatives, hypnotics and narcotics) provide some measure of cerebral protection, but in the absence of reversible factors, attempts to resuscitate a patient from non-VF/VT arrest should be terminated after 20 minutes.

Should relatives be allowed to watch resuscitation attempts?

In many emergency departments and medical admission units it has become standard practice to allow relatives to observe resuscitation. The presence of family members during resuscitation efforts has been shown to aid the grieving process should resuscitation prove unsuccessful, but families should not be encouraged to enter the resuscitation room if they are reluctant.

> ⚠ Relatives should only be allowed to observe resuscitation if there is a trained member of staff present whose sole responsibility is to support them. To have relatives watching with no one to explain what is going on and attend to their needs is asking for trouble.

1.2.2 Chest pain and hypotension

Scenario

A 48-year-old male taxi driver has been brought into the Emergency Department. He is complaining of chest pain and breathlessness. He has a pulse rate of 130 bpm and his BP is 80/40 mmHg. You are asked to see him urgently by the nurse in charge.

Introduction

> 🔑 In dealing with a patient who is very ill, resuscitation should begin immediately and history-taking, examination and investigation should be concurrent. To start by trying to take a detailed history from someone who is dying is likely to end in death and is not good medicine!

TABLE 1 DIFFERENTIAL DIAGNOSIS OF HYPOTENSIVE COLLAPSE

Common	Must consider	Other causes
Cardiovascular catastrophe: myocardial infarction, pulmonary embolism Hypovolaemia, particularly gastrointestinal blood loss Surgical cause: ruptured abdominal aortic aneurysm or a perforated viscus Sepsis: pneumonia and septicaemia	Aortic dissection Tension pneumothorax Fluid loss from other causes, eg profound diarrhoea in an elderly person living alone Multiple problems, particularly in the elderly (eg acute viral infection, inadequate fluid intake and complicating myocardial infarction)	Addisonian crisis Hypothermia or hypothyroidism Cardiac tamponade

Priorities

- Resuscitation: airway, breathing and circulation (ABC).

- Try to establish a diagnosis (Table 1).

Resuscitation

Regardless of the specific diagnosis, your priorities must be to correct any problem with airway, breathing or circulation.

> 🔑 Get help early for any patient who is extremely unwell. Don't worry about establishing a diagnosis: ask for senior assistance. If necessary, put out a cardiac arrest call: it is much better to get the arrest team there to help than to wait until the patient's heart has stopped.

Airway/breathing Ensure the patient's airway is patent: consider the placement of a nasopharyngeal or oropharyngeal airway if conscious level is depressed. Apply an oxygen saturation monitor. Give high-flow oxygen. If the patient does not respond promptly to this or is ventilating inadequately, then intubation and ventilation may be required. Call for anaesthetic assistance sooner rather than later.

> ⚠ **Hypoxia kills, hypercapnia merely intoxicates**
>
> Even patients with known chronic obstructive pulmonary disease should receive high-flow oxygen if they are *in extremis*. The oxygen may buy you enough time to institute other treatments and the patient can then be slowly weaned from it according to blood gas analysis.

Circulation Two large (grey) venflons should be inserted into the antecubital fossae. If you are confident that a patient is hypovolaemic (exceedingly unlikely in this case), then give intravenous fluids quickly to the hypotensive patient until the circulation is restored. In most cases 0.9% (normal) saline will be appropriate initially. If there is evidence of acute blood loss, then blood should be transfused: an emergency cross-match should be available within 20–30 minutes, but if fluid replacement is more urgent than this then colloid solutions can be given (or O negative blood).

> 🔑 Resuscitation should be swift! There is no merit in resuscitating more slowly than is possible.

> **Fluid resuscitation of the hypovolaemic patient**
>
> - Give 0.5 L of 0.9% saline as fast as possible.
> - Recheck peripheral perfusion, pulse, BP and JVP.
> - If still hypovolaemic, give further 0.5 L of 0.9% saline as fast as possible.
> - Repeat cycle until signs of hypovolaemia are corrected.

Insert a urinary catheter to monitor fluid output. The urinary catheter is the poor man's central venous pressure (CVP) line and allows measurement of organ perfusion. A urine output of 50 mL/hour suggests that renal perfusion is adequate.

Central venous cannulation in the neck should not be attempted at this stage. It is difficult to access the internal jugular or subclavian vein in a patient who is breathless and cannot lie flat or who is hypovolaemic, and iatrogenic pneumothorax or haemothorax is also not a good idea (Fig. 3). If peripheral access cannot be achieved, insert a femoral line (see Section 1.2.15).

> ⚠ Never try to insert an internal jugular or subclavian venous line into a patient who is obviously hypovolaemic.

> ⚠
> - A 'normal' CVP reading does not necessarily mean that the patient would not benefit from more fluid.
> - Right-sided cardiac pressures reveal only part of the picture: it is possible to have a normal or high right atrial pressure at a time when left ventricular filling is inadequate, eg with major pulmonary embolism (PE). If in doubt, give a fluid bolus of 250 mL and observe the response carefully.

If the patient remains hypotensive when intravascular volume has been restored, consider the following.

- An additional fluid challenge: however, do not induce fluid overload and pulmonary oedema, which would be the almost certain outcome of a fluid challenge in this scenario.

- Inotropes: these can be used if there is circulatory pump failure. Vasoconstricting drugs may be necessary if vasodilatation is part of the pathological process, eg sepsis.

However, before escalating treatment in this way, the appropriateness of intensive care for the individual patient must be discussed and ratified (see Section 1.1.3).

> **Management of the hypotensive patient**
>
> - Ensure airway, breathing and circulation are all satisfactory.
> - Give high-flow oxygen.
> - Check if patient is hypovolaemic. Is there another reason for the hypotension?
> - If hypovolaemic, give the correct fluid quickly.
> - Is specific treatment indicated for the particular primary pathology?
> - If still hypotensive, proceed to invasive haemodynamic measurement, inotropic and/or vasoconstricting drugs as indicated.

History of the presenting problem

Chest pain

- Dull, crushing, central chest pain radiating to the neck or arms in association with nausea, vomiting, pallor and sweating would suggest a primary cardiac cause.

- The chest pain associated with PE may be dull or pleuritic.

- Sharp tearing chest pain radiating to the back may indicate a dissecting aortic aneurysm.

- Could this be pain coming from an abdominal pathology?

Breathlessness

- Did the breathlessness come on suddenly or gradually? Sudden

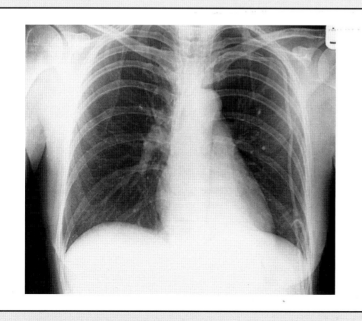

▲ **Fig. 3** Left subclavian line and iatrogenic left pneumothorax.

MMC Core Curriculum   **13**

onset (in an instant) suggests pneumothorax, large airway obstruction or PE. Is there any suggestion that the patient has had multiple small PEs?

- Has the patient suffered from orthopnoea or paroxysmal nocturnal dyspnoea? These would suggest pulmonary oedema, but be aware that a patient with any cause of breathlessness will not want to lie down.

Any other features?

- Has the patient been feverish or systemically unwell? Could he have a severe pneumonia?

- Has the patient had leg pain or swelling, or had haemoptysis? These would clearly point towards PE in this context.

Other relevant history

It will clearly be important to find out if the patient has previously had problems with angina or myocardial infarction, or (much less likely) any of the other diagnoses listed in Table 1. If he says 'the pain is just like when I had a heart attack last year', then the diagnosis is almost made.

Examination

> When assessing patients who present acutely, the first thing to do is to decide whether they are well, ill, very ill or nearly dead: it is vital for appropriate management to decide quickly which category they are in.

Overall assessment of the adequacy of the cardiovascular system

- If cardiac output is impaired, there is often a marked cut-off peripherally between warm dry skin and a cold clammy feel. Run your hand down the patient's arm,

starting from the shoulder, and observe where the change occurs. Patients who are septic have a high cardiac output with low systemic resistance, such that they are peripherally vasodilated with warm sweaty skin.

- Check the capillary return by pressing on the nail-bed to blanch it and then measuring the time taken for the colour to return on releasing the pressure: normally it should be less than 2 seconds; more than 5 seconds is clearly abnormal.

- Heart rate and rhythm, BP when lying and standing (or sitting, if the patient is too unwell to stand), and height of the JVP should always be measured. Measure the JVP in centimetres from the angle of Louis, angling the patient up or down until venous pulsation is seen: it is not good enough to settle for 'venous pressure not elevated'.

- Simple measures of organ perfusion include the ability of the patient to respond to questioning and the amount of urine produced per hour.

Cardiovascular

In addition to assessing the overall adequacy of the cardiovascular system, check carefully for the following when performing the cardiovascular examination.

- Can you feel the left radial pulse as well as the right? If it seems to be diminished, measure BP in both arms and consider aortic dissection.

- Can you hear any murmurs? Acute mitral valve regurgitation or a ventricular septal defect can complicate an acute myocardial infarction and cause catastrophic heart failure (see *Cardiology*, Section 1.4.4). Always consider the possibility of bacterial endocarditis when a murmur is discovered (see *Cardiology*, Sections 1.4.7 and 2.8.1).

- Consider PE: look for leg swelling, elevated JVP, right ventricular heave, right ventricular gallop and loud P2.

- Consider pericardial effusion: it is easy to overlook this possibility (Fig. 4), but the signs of pulsus

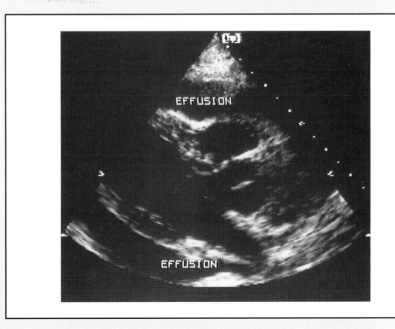

▲**Fig. 4** Echocardiogram of a large pericardial effusion.

paradoxus (exaggeration of the normal fall in systolic BP that occurs on inspiration to >10 mmHg, which must be measured with a sphygmomanometer) and elevation of the venous pressure with inspiration (Kussmaul's sign) should be part of your routine examination (see *Cardiology*, Sections 2.6.2 and 2.6.3).

Respiratory

A tension pneumothorax can present with circulatory collapse or cardiac arrest, so look specifically for the following.

- The chest often looks asymmetrical, with the affected side 'blown up'.
- The trachea is deviated away from the affected side.
- The mediastinum is shifted away from the affected side, which can be detected by finding displacement of the apex beat or shift of the area of cardiac dullness on percussion.
- The affected side of the chest is silent.

In this case it would be much more likely that you would hear the crackles of pulmonary oedema, but look also for signs that might indicate pneumonic consolidation (dullness to percussion and bronchial breathing) or a pleural rub (consistent with PE or pneumonia).

Abdominal

A number of abdominal pathologies can cause collapse with or without chest pain. Check for abdominal distension, bruising in the flanks, aortic aneurysm (palpate deliberately in the epigastrium), herniae and peritonism. Consider the following diagnoses: ruptured abdominal aortic aneurysm, perforated viscus, pancreatitis, cholecystitis/cholangitis and intestinal obstruction.

⚠ **Coma and hypotension: which came first, the chicken or the egg?**

If a patient who is unconscious is also hypotensive, it is far more likely that the hypotension is the cause of the unconsciousness than vice versa. Primary intracerebral pathologies that result in hypotension are rare; hypotension causing inadequate cerebral perfusion is common.

Investigation

Tests to be requested immediately in the Emergency Department include the following.

- Pulse oximetery; fingerprick blood glucose.

- ECG: look in particular at rate/rhythm (is the pulse of 130 bpm sinus rhythm or an arrhythmia that might benefit from treatment?) and for evidence of myocardial infarction.

- Routine blood tests: FBC, electrolytes, renal/liver/bone profile, clotting and troponin.

- Cultures: blood, urine and cerebrospinal fluid as indicated.

- Arterial blood gases: pulse oximetry can be unreliable in patients who are hypotensive. Measurement of arterial blood gases is essential to check oxygen tension and pH.

- CXR: this may give vital information. A widened mediastinum or evidence of air under the diaphragm may reveal the diagnosis.

- Other investigations: as determined by clinical suspicion, eg CT angiogram for aortic dissection (see Section 1.2.3) or CT pulmonary angiogram for PE (see Section 1.2.10).

Management

In addition to resuscitation described above, also consider the following.

Antibiotics

If there is a possibility of sepsis as a diagnosis, then prescribe broad-spectrum antibiotics. The choice will depend on the likely source, the local prevalence of organisms, recent travel and previous antibiotic exposure. Involve the microbiologist as early as possible. Remember that sepsis can present atypically and always take blood cultures before prescribing antibiotics.

Other specific conditions

Any of the conditions listed in Table 1 will require rapid specific treatment.

- Myocardial infarction: clearly the most likely diagnosis in this case (see *Cardiology*, Section 1.4.3 and 2.1.3).

- PE: see *Cardiology*, Sections 1.4.6 and 2.18.1.

- Tension pneumothorax: see Section 1.2.12.

- Gastrointestinal haemorrhage: see *Gastroenterology and Hepatology*, Section 1.4.3.

- Intra-abdominal catastrophe: arrange for urgent surgical consultation if the main problem seems to be abdominal.

1.2.3 Should he be thrombolysed?

Scenario

A 57-year-old businessman presents to the Emergency Department with a history of severe central crushing chest pain of 1 hour's duration. This followed a stressful business meeting. The nurse in charge asks you whether he should have thrombolytic therapy.

Introduction

> ⚠️ Between 2 and 4% of patients with an acute myocardial infarction are discharged inappropriately from the Emergency Department. This is more likely to occur in women than men, and also in the elderly and non-white people.

The most likely diagnosis is acute coronary syndrome (ACS). Immediate priorities are as follows.

Resuscitation and immediate assessment

- Airway, breathing and circulation (ABC).

- Administer high-flow oxygen and apply a saturation monitor.

- Check the heart rate and rhythm. Feel for pulses and check the BP in both arms. Check peripheral perfusion (see Section 1.2.2). Obtain intravenous access.

- All patients with possible ACS should have continuous cardiac monitoring because cardiac arrhythmias are common in this condition and need prompt treatment.

Diagnosis

Look carefully at the ECG: if it is diagnostic for ST-elevation acute myocardial infarction (STEMI), then consider reperfusion therapy immediately.

> 🔑 **ECG criteria for STEMI**
> - 1 mm or more ST-segment elevation in two or more standard ECG leads.
> - 2 mm or more ST-segment elevation in two or more contiguous precordial leads (in typical infarct pattern).
> - New left bundle branch block.

History of the presenting problem

Look for features in the history to suggest that this patient is suffering from an ACS.

- Patients with more severe pain are more likely to have an ACS, but be wary: social, professional and age-related differences influence the presentation of symptoms. Women are more likely to complain of referred pain to the neck, jaw and back.

- Ischaemic pain is more likely to be diffuse and of longer duration. The pain of an acute myocardial infarction (AMI) is likely to be described as a constant pressure and may be associated with sweating, nausea and vomiting.

Other relevant history

The current American Heart Association/American College of Cardiology guidelines recommend that five factors should be considered together when assessing the likelihood of myocardial ischaemia relating to ACS.

1. Nature of the symptoms: high-risk factors include worsening angina, prolonged pain (>20 minutes), pulmonary oedema, hypotension and arrhythmias.

2. History of ischaemic heart disease: has the patient any known history of previous angina/AMI or had any symptoms to suggest such a diagnosis, which might not have been recognised previously?

3. Age.

4. Sex.

5. Number of traditional cardiac risk factors present, including a positive family history, known hypertension, hypercholesterolaemia, diabetes and smoking.

Examination

Attention will clearly focus on cardiac and respiratory examination, but look for the following features that would suggest a diagnosis of ACS.

- The patient with ischaemic pain is likely to have autonomic signs and may be sweating, clammy, cool and pale.

- AMI is more likely if the patient has hypotension and a third heart sound.

- Exclusion of other diagnoses: check peripheral pulses to rule out aortic dissection; listen for murmurs and pericardial or pleural rubs.

Investigation

ECG

This is clearly the most important initial investigation in this case: look carefully for any signs of STEMI (Fig. 5) and act on it immediately. Around one-third of patients with an AMI will not have ST elevation on arrival: look for ST depression, T-wave inversion, Q waves or any conduction defect. If the ECG is normal on arrival and the clinical suspicion is high, then arrange for serial ECGs. The sensitivity of the initial ECG is said to be as low as 50%. The number of patients eligible for thrombolysis can be increased by extending the lateral leads further across the chest (V7–9) and by applying right-sided chest leads (rV1–6).

Look also for features of pericarditis, when the typical ECG changes are of peaked 'T' waves and ST segments which are elevated and concave upwards. However, there is another appearance that can help with the diagnosis: the isoelectric line on the ECG is the TP interval and in those with acute pericarditis

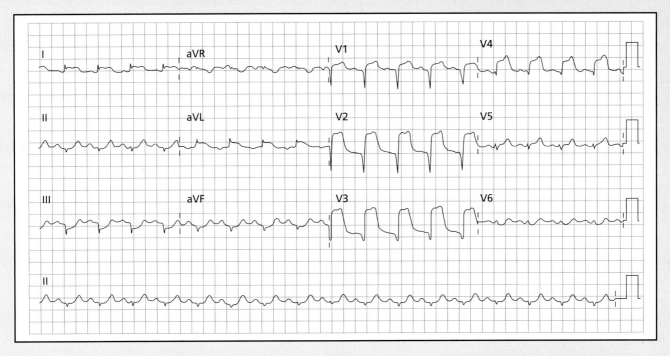

▲**Fig. 5** ECG of acute anterior myocardial infarction with early Q-wave formation.

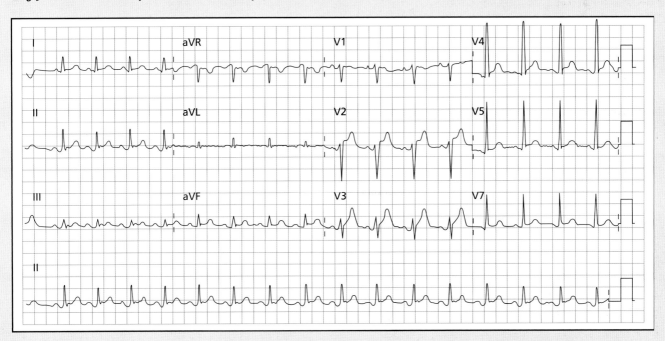

▲**Fig. 6** ECG of acute pericarditis: the ST-segment changes are obvious but note also the depressed PR interval shown especially in leads II and aVF.

there is sometimes depression of the following PR interval (Fig. 6).

Blood tests

- Troponin(s).

- Electrolytes.

- Renal and liver function tests.

- Blood sugar.

- Lipid levels.

- FBC and clotting.

Chest radiograph

Measure heart size, exclude pulmonary oedema and look for the widened mediastinum of aortic dissection.

Management of unstable angina/non-ST-elevation myocardial infarction

General

- Oxygen, cardiac monitoring and pain relief with opioids.

- Sublingual nitrates, and consider intravenous or buccal nitrates if pain recurs.

- Assess for complications such as left ventricular failure and tachyarrhythmias.

Antiplatelet therapy

- Aspirin: all patients thought to have ACS should be given 300 mg aspirin and then continued on 75 mg daily.

- Clopidogrel: start clopidogrel in patients presenting with ACS and continue treatment for up to 12 months.

- Glycoprotein IIb/IIIa inhibitors (eg tirofiban): give these in high-risk patients. The definition of this category varies from centre to centre, but is commonly (i) those patients who have unstable symptoms with positive troponin assay, (ii) those patients who meet the criteria as defined according to the Thrombolysis In Myocardial Infarction (TIMI) risk score (see below) or particularly (iii) those in whom percutaneous coronary intervention is planned.

TIMI risk score

Risk factors
Each risk factor scores 1 point

1. Age >65 years
2. More than three risk factors (family history, hypertension, hypercholesterolaemia, diabetes mellitus and smoking) for coronary artery disease
3. Known coronary artery disease (stenosis >50%)
4. Aspirin use in the past 7 days

Presentation
Each presentation scores 1 point
5. Recent severe angina (<24 hours)
6. Raised cardiac markers
7. ST-segment change >0.5 mm

Risk score
- Total points = 7
- High risk, score >3

Anticoagulant therapy

Low-molecular-weight heparin reduces the risk of myocardial infarction and increases the rate of reperfusion compared with unfractionated heparin.

Other treatments

- β-Adrenoceptor blockade: start this, unless contraindicated, as first-line antianginal therapy. Consider diltiazem if beta-blockers are contraindicated, but avoid dihydropyridine calcium channel blockers (eg nifedipine).

- Statins and angiotensin-converting enzyme (ACE) inhibitors: start in all patients with positive cardiac markers if not already on them and there are no contraindications.

Management of ST-elevation myocardial infarction

General

- Provide oxygen, cardiac monitoring and pain relief with opioids.

- Assess for complications such as left ventricular failure and tachyarrhythmias.

Reperfusion therapy

Maximum benefit is seen when this is started within 1 hour of symptoms. Reperfusion can be achieved by either primary percutaneous coronary intervention (PCI) or thrombolytic therapy. Primary PCI is the recommended method, but its major limitation is that it requires 24-hour availability of a staffed catheter laboratory and a skilled operator. In the many circumstances where PCI is not available, thrombolytic therapy has been shown to provide substantial reduction in mortality from AMI when given in the first few hours after the onset of chest pain.

If there are no contraindications to thrombolysis (see below), then a tissue-type plasminogen activator is the agent of choice, particularly for anterior myocardial infarction when symptoms have been present for less than 4 hours. A tissue-type plasminogen activator should always be used if streptokinase has been administered previously and in patients whose systolic BP is less than 100 mmHg.

Contraindications to thrombolysis

- Cerebrovascular accident/peptic ulcer/gastrointestinal bleed within the preceding 3 months.
- Surgery or trauma within the preceding 2 weeks.
- BP more than 200/110 mmHg.
- Bleeding diathesis.
- Structural cerebrovascular lesions, including neoplasms.
- History of intracerebral haemorrhage.
- Aortic dissection.

Patients presenting with STEMI within 6 hours of symptom onset and who fail to reperfuse following thrombolysis should undergo rescue PCI.

Antiplatelet therapy

- Aspirin: all patients with ACS should be given 300 mg aspirin and then continued on 75 mg daily.

- Clopidogrel: start clopidogrel in patients presenting with ACS, and continue treatment for up to 12 months.

Other treatments

- Insulin: give intravenous insulin for diabetics or in patients whose blood glucose is >11 mmol/L.

- β-Adrenoceptor blockade: start this, unless contraindicated, and continue indefinitely.

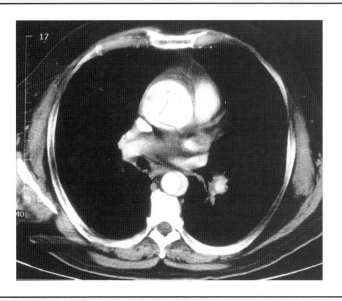

▲**Fig. 7** Mediastinal CT scan showing the classical appearances of aortic dissection: note the 'tennis-ball' appearance of the ascending and descending aorta.

Pericarditis

A therapeutic trial of aspirin or other NSAIDs can sometimes help in diagnosing pericarditis; relief of pericarditic pain commonly occurs within 20 minutes (see *Cardiology*, Sections 1.4.8 and 2.6.1).

Oesophageal pain

Inevitably, there will be some situations in which it is impossible to decide between an oesophageal and a cardiac aetiology. In these situations, your fall-back position must be to consider it cardiac until proved otherwise.

- Statins and ACE inhibitors: start these in all patients if not already on them and there are no contraindications.

Further comments

Patients with negative cardiac markers (no elevation of troponin) and those with a TIMI score <2 have been shown not to benefit from an early invasive strategy. They need assessment prior to discharge based on their cardiac risk and current symptoms. This will depend on local resources. Early exercise testing may be of value in those with suspected angina but without a definite history of preceding angina of effort or myocardial infarction, and also without high-risk features on presentation and a negative troponin at 6–8 hours. Others may require outpatient follow-up including stress testing.

Two-dimensional echocardiography can identify regional wall abnormalities in patients with cardiac ischaemia and may also detect important prognostic information such as systolic dysfunction.

Aortic dissection

If dissection is suspected, the definitive investigations are either CT (Fig. 7) or transoesophageal echocardiography (Fig. 8). Surgery should be considered urgently for patients with proximal aortic dissection.

Diagnostic uncertainty

If you do not know the diagnosis, be honest with yourself and with the patient. It does not mean that you have 'failed': the diagnosis may be impossible to make. Consider the major diagnoses discussed. Therapeutic trials may give aid diagnostically, but the default position must be to consider the most serious potential conditions and treat them appropriately until further evidence has secured the diagnosis.

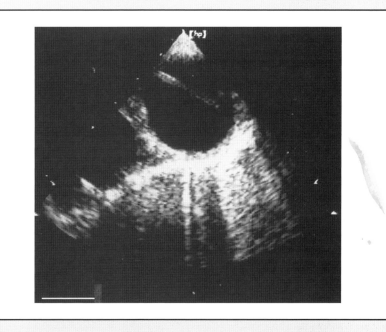

▲**Fig. 8** Transoesophageal echocardiogram showing the flap of dissection in the aorta.

1.2.4 Hypotension in acute coronary syndrome

Scenario

A 72-year-old man is admitted to the coronary care unit with chest pain. He has known ischaemic heart disease and has had previous coronary artery bypass grafts. On presentation he was sweaty, with BP 120/70 mmHg and a clear chest. His ECG on arrival in the Emergency Department showed ST-segment depression and T-wave changes inferiorly. He was commenced on maximal medical therapy, including aspirin, intravenous nitrates, intravenous beta-blockers, low-molecular-weight heparin and clopidogrel. It is now 6 hours since his admission: he has become drowsy and his BP has fallen to 70/50 mmHg. You are bleeped to review him urgently.

Introduction

The cause of profound hypotension in a patient with an acute coronary syndrome can usually be established by examining the patient, obtaining an ECG and CXR, and review of the drug chart.

🔑 **Check airway, breathing and circulation, and begin management immediately.**

- Administer high-flow oxygen and monitor pulse oximetry.
- Check heart rate and rhythm, and the BP in both arms.
- Obtain intravenous access (if not already established).
- Give 250 mL fluid bolus if the chest is clear.
- Stop any drugs that may be contributing to hypotension.
- Call for help early.

History of the presenting problem

This man is unlikely to respond well to attempts to take a lengthy history from him, but important things to find out, from him and from scrutiny of the observation charts, include the following.

- Is he in pain? Ongoing or new pain in an acute coronary syndrome may indicate development of ST-elevation myocardial infarction (in other words, an acute myocardial infarction, AMI), or cardiac rupture.

- Has his BP fallen suddenly or gradually? A sudden onset of low BP in association with new chest pain is again suggestive of cardiac rupture. Low BP in association with breathlessness resulting from left ventricular pump failure tends to be more gradual in onset.

- What drugs has he been given? Look closely for a temporal relationship between his hypotension and the administration of drugs. Although not applicable in this case, hypotension during infusion of streptokinase is common and usually occurs during the first 20 minutes.

Examination

Key features to concentrate on include the following.

- Peripheral perfusion: it is a poor prognostic sign if the patient is shut down. How far up the arms and legs is he cold?

- Heart rate and rhythm: could a secondary tachycardia or bradycardia be the cause of hypotension?

- BP in both arms: could the patient have had an aortic dissection in association with an inferior myocardial infarction?

- JVP: if this is markedly raised, consider right ventricular infarction, ventricular septal defect (VSD), tamponade or pulmonary embolism. A low JVP would be a surprise in this clinical context, but if found consider the possibility of gastrointestinal bleeding, especially if thrombolysis has been given.

- Auscultation of the heart: a new pansystolic murmur would suggest a VSD or mitral regurgitation as a result of chordal or papillary muscle rupture; a gallop rhythm would be expected.

- Crackles in the chest, indicating pulmonary oedema.

- Pulse oximetry.

Quantitate the patient's 'drowsiness' by checking his score on the Glasgow Coma Scale. Depression of consciousness may be due to hypotension, opioids (how much morphine has he had? Are pupils pinpoint? If so, give naloxone) or, particularly if thrombolysis has been given, stroke (look for deviation of gaze, facial asymmetry and hemiparesis).

Investigation

See Sections 1.2.2 and 1.2.3 for fuller discussion, but the following are clearly vital in this case.

- ECG: repeat to assess cardiac rhythm and look for evidence of ongoing ischaemia. In particular, has an inferior infarct pattern developed and are there signs of right ventricular infarction?

- CXR: will give some information about pre-existing chest and cardiac conditions (cardiac shape and size) as well as an assessment of pulmonary congestion.

- Echocardiogram: likely to be the most useful investigation in this case, particularly for detecting acute mitral regurgitation, VSD and tamponade, and also in enabling assessment of global overall right and left ventricular function and focal abnormalities thereof.

Management

Again see Sections 1.2.2 and 1.2.3 for fuller discussion, but note the following particularly relevant to this case.

> Has anyone spoken to the relatives and informed them of what has happened? This man is desperately ill and may die soon.

General supportive measures

- High-flow oxygen and respiratory support with the aim of maximising oxygen delivery. Use of continuous positive airway pressure may decrease intubation rates, but no decrease in mortality has yet been shown. Consider intubation if there is acute respiratory failure which is not responding to medical treatment.

- Analgesia: if the patient is in pain do not withhold adequate analgesia, but give small doses at a time (eg morphine 2.5 mg iv, with antiemetic).

- Fluids: the hypotensive hypoxic patient with bilateral crackles will not respond well to a fluid challenge, but give a cautious fluid bolus (250 mL) if hypotensive with a clear chest, even with a raised JVP. In the setting of an inferior myocardial infarction this could reflect right ventricular ischaemia and volume loading alone may improve the cardiac output.

- Monitoring: haemodynamically unstable patients need close monitoring. Central venous pressure lines have a role, but be cautious with the readings, watch the trend and do not over-interpret. Do not underestimate the value of a urinary catheter and measurement of hourly urine output in assessment of the circulation.

Other methods of circulatory support

- Inotropes: evidence for their benefit is limited. They can obviously raise the arterial pressure, which looks better on the observation charts, but there is no compelling evidence that they improve prognosis. The resulting high systemic vascular resistance means they should be used with caution and for a limited time only because they can lead to a further decrease in end-organ tissue perfusion.

- Intra-aortic balloon counterpulsation: another holding method whose use should be restricted to patients with an underlying condition that (i) can be treated, with percutaneous coronary intervention (PCI), valve replacement, repair of VSD or (not appropriate in this case) heart transplant, or (ii) that will recover spontaneously (early post AMI, or post surgery or myocarditis).

Specific measures

Specialist advice is needed: would this man benefit from PCI, valve replacement or repair of VSD?

> If there are no obvious reversible or treatable factors and no satisfactory response to initial medical treatment, then palliation of symptoms must be the priority.

1.2.5 Postoperative breathlessness

Scenario

You are the duty medical doctor and are called to see a 71-year-old man on a surgical ward at 3 a.m. He is complaining of breathlessness. The nursing staff report that his saturations remain persistently low and he is deteriorating despite increasing amounts of oxygen. He has a past history of ischaemic heart disease, hypertension and a smoking history of 30 pack-years.

Introduction

Three diagnoses are likely: chest infection/pneumonia/exacerbation of chronic obstructive pulmonary disease (COPD); pulmonary oedema; or pulmonary embolism (PE). You will obviously begin by making a rapid assessment of the severity of the man's condition and initiating any immediate treatment that is required (see Section 1.2.2), but bear these conditions in mind as you take the history and examine the patient.

History of the presenting problem

Look at the medical and nursing records

Why is the man in hospital and what (if any) surgery has he had?

- If he had surgery, was this complicated by significant blood loss or hypovolaemia, which may have precipitated myocardial infarction (MI) and thereby pulmonary oedema in this man with known ischaemic heart disease?

- Do the medical and nursing records suggest that the man has been 'going off' for some days, or does this seem to be an acute event?

- Look at his fluid balance chart: is he in a significant positive balance that would explain pulmonary oedema, perhaps because of the development of perioperative acute renal failure?

- Look carefully at his drug chart and compare this with the medications he was taking on admission: have any drugs, for instance diuretics or bronchodilators, been stopped (probably inadvertently) on admission that might explain his deterioration?

- Review laboratory records: has his serum creatinine risen postoperatively to indicate that he has acute renal failure?

> When assessing any patient who has deteriorated in hospital, always look carefully through the medical, nursing and laboratory records.

Symptoms suggesting pulmonary oedema

Has the man had any ischaemic cardiac chest pain or been aware of any palpitations? Angina, MI or transient tachyarrhythmia could all compromise left ventricular function and precipitate pulmonary oedema.

Symptoms suggesting PE

Ask specifically about leg pain or swelling, pleuritic chest pain or haemoptysis.

Symptoms suggesting chest infection/pneumonia/exacerbation of COPD

These diagnoses would be supported by a history of nausea or vomiting, or the presence of a nasogastric tube, all of which increase risk of aspiration. High fever (>38.5°C) would support the diagnosis, but remember there may be many causes for fever in a postoperative patient, and also that MI and PE typically cause low-grade fever. Pleuritic chest pain could be due to pneumonia (and also PE, as stated above). Wheezing supports the diagnosis of COPD, but can also be caused by pulmonary oedema.

Examination

An immediate assessment of the severity of the illness is required: is the patient ill, very ill or nearly dead? Look for the features described in Section 1.2.2, noting in particular the following.

Cardiovascular

- Heart rate and rhythm: sinus tachycardia is likely to be present, but check for the presence of an arrhythmia (of which atrial fibrillation would be the most likely).

- BP and peripheral perfusion: significant cardiac compromise will result in a low-output state with hypotension and poor peripheral perfusion (capillary refill >5 seconds). Pulsus alternans (alternation between large- and low-volume pulse) may also be a sign in severe left ventricular failure.

- JVP: an elevated venous pressure could be due to heart failure or PE in this context, but it can be very difficult to identify the JVP in someone who is hyperventilating and frightened.

- Added heart sounds and murmurs: these may suggest a primary cardiac pathology, although by themselves they do not secure the diagnosis. In pulmonary oedema a 'gallop rhythm' with the addition of a third heart sound may be heard. Features of PE can include a third heart sound over the right ventricle and a loud P2.

Respiratory

Dullness to percussion may indicate lung consolidation or pleural effusion. Wheezes may be due to pulmonary oedema ('cardiac asthma') or COPD in this man. Pulmonary crepitations/ crackles, particularly if bibasal, suggest pulmonary oedema. A pleural rub would be consistent with PE or pneumonia.

Other systems

Establish a baseline for higher cerebral function (Abbreviated Mental Test Score) and neurological state (Glasgow Coma Scale). Examine the patient's abdomen. Is there acute urinary obstruction with a large tender bladder? Has he had an intra-abdominal catastrophe manifest with distension and/or peritonism?

Investigation

The following are required urgently.

- ECG: to exclude an acute or previous MI, look for evidence of myocardial ischaemia and assess the heart rhythm. These may occasionally show features (manifestations of right ventricular strain) to support a diagnosis of PE, but these are not reliable for confirming or refuting this diagnosis.

- CXR: left ventricular failure will classically produce bilateral alveolar/interstitial shadowing, 'batwing' perihilar shadowing, fluid within the horizontal fissure, bilateral pleural effusions and cardiomegaly (Fig. 9). Pneumonia will typically show consolidation.

Other tests in all patients with this presentation include the following.

- FBC to rule out significant anaemia.

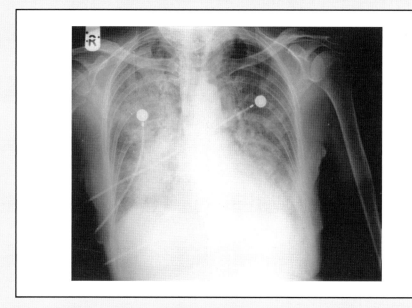

▲ **Fig. 9** CXR showing features of severe left ventricular failure.

- Electrolytes and renal function: acute renal failure and iatrogenic fluid overload may explain pulmonary oedema.

- Troponin I/T (immediately and 12 hours following any acute event) as marker of myocardial damage: but note that minor elevation is not specific for MI.

- Arterial blood gases: to assess oxgenation, ventilation and acidosis in any patient who is very unwell.

Other tests depend on clinical suspicion. If PE is suspected, then CT pulmonary angiography is the investigation of choice in this context (when a ventilation–perfusion scan is not likely to be interpretable). If an infective cause is expected, then take blood and sputum (if available) cultures. Note that echocardiography is increasingly available as an emergency investigation and can be particularly helpful in assessing left ventricular function, but interpret it with caution in patients with tachyarrhythmias.

Management

Immediate priorities

- Airway, breathing and circulation (ABC).

- Administer high-flow oxygen.

- Sit the patient up.

- Apply ECG monitoring and peripheral oxygen saturation monitoring.

- Obtain venous access.

- Organise the investigations listed above.

Specific treatment will depend on the diagnosis: for PE see Section 1.2.8; for pneumonia see Section 1.2.11; for exacerbation of COPD see Section 1.2.10.

Pulmonary oedema

For pulmonary oedema give diuretics (eg furosemide 40–80 mg iv), sublingual nitrates or an intravenous nitrate infusion, and a low dose of opioid (eg diamorphine 2.5 mg iv, with antiemetic). Call for help if the patient does not improve

rapidly: he may need non-invasive or invasive ventilation (see Section 3.8).

Consider reasons why the patient may have developed pulmonary oedema/acute left ventricular failure. Are there any heart murmurs? If so, request an urgent echocardiogram: acute mitral regurgitation and ventricular septal defect are both complications of MI (Fig. 10). Does a repeated ECG show evidence of evolving MI?

1.2.6 Two patients with tachyarrhythmia

Scenario

You are called to the medical assessment unit where two patients have arrived at the same time. They are both tachycardic. The first is a 72-year-old woman with chest pain, and the second is a woman of 25 years complaining of palpitations. Which patient should you deal with first?

Introduction

Some arrhythmias left untreated can cause cardiac arrest, whereas others may need no immediate treatment. You need to be able to recognise common arrhythmias in order to know which need immediate treatment.

Adverse features of tachyarrhythmias

- Systolic BP <90 mmHg.
- Heart rate >150 bpm.
- Chest pain.
- Heart failure.
- Drowsiness or confusion.

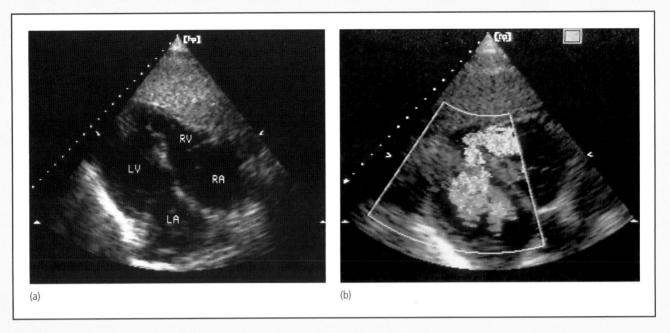

(a)

(b)

▲**Fig. 10** Echocardiogram of a ventricular septal defect following MI (**a**) and the flow across the defect (**b**). LA, left atrium; LV, left ventricle; RA, right atrium; RV, right ventricle.

> **Management of a tachyarrhythmia associated with adverse features should include the following.**
>
> - Call for help immediately.
> - Give high-flow oxygen.
> - Apply cardiac monitor.
> - Insert intravenous access.
> - Prepare for synchronised cardioversion immediately, with sedation or a general anaesthetic.

History of the presenting problem

The risks of coronary artery disease and myocardial ischaemia increase with age. Ventricular tachycardia (VT) is far more likely in someone who has known coronary artery disease or has had a previous acute myocardial infarction (AMI).

Other relevant history

Obtain the old notes: old ECGs are invaluable. Is there evidence of an innate electrical abnormality, eg classical accessory pathways of the Wolff–Parkinson–White (WPW) or Lown–Ganong–Levine syndromes?

Look for an echocardiogram result: what was the left ventricular function and was there evidence of structural heart problems (eg valve disease or cardiomyopathy)?

Examination

An overall assessment of the adequacy of the cardiovascular system is required, as described in Section 1.2.2. If the arrhythmia is not well tolerated the heart may start to fail as cardiac output falls; if there is inadequate time in diastole for cardiac filling the myocardium becomes ischaemic, which will be worse if there is underlying coronary artery disease. These clinical features will dictate the speed at which treatment is needed.

Investigation

After checking for clinical features that would indicate adverse prognosis, obtain a 12-lead ECG immediately.

Is this a broad- or narrow-complex tachycardia?

Are the QRS complexes narrow (<120 ms) or broad (>120 ms)?

Broad-complex tachycardias tend to be less well tolerated because there is often underlying heart disease. If in doubt, always assume a broad-complex tachycardia is a VT until proved otherwise. The use of verapamil to treat VT could cause severe and prolonged hypotension or even cardiac arrest; in contrast, attempts to correct a VT are unlikely to cause any further compromise in a supraventricular tachycardia (SVT).

> **Assume a broad-complex tachycardia is a VT until proved otherwise.**

Is a broad-complex tachycardia a VT or an SVT with aberrant conduction?

VT is more likely if the following are present.

- Atrioventricular (AV) dissociation: more QRS complexes than P waves is diagnostic of VT.

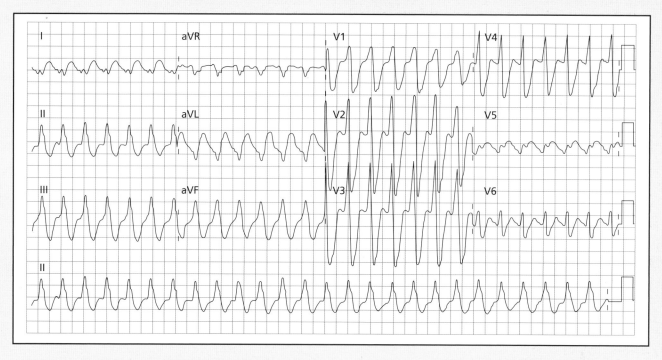

▲ **Fig. 11** Ventricular tachycardia showing wide QRS complexes and concordance.

- Very wide QRS complexes: the wider the complexes, the more likely that the origin of the arrhythmia is ventricular (Fig. 11). QRS complexes >0.14 seconds wide are almost 100% certain to be due to VT.

- Capture beats and fusion beats.

- Concordance: the phenomenon where QRS complexes have the same morphology across all the chest leads.

- Extreme left-axis deviation or a change in axis from an old ECG.

An irregular broad-complex tachycardia could be atrial fibrillation with bundle branch block or, less commonly, atrial fibrillation with ventricular pre-excitation. Polymorphic VT (torsade de pointes) is another possibility, but remember that this is unusual without any adverse features.

Regular narrow-complex tachycardias

- Sinus tachycardia.

- AV nodal re-entry tachycardia: the commonest type of SVT.

- AV re-entrant tachycardia: pre-excitation including WPW syndrome.

- Atrial flutter with regular AV conduction (usually 2:1) (Fig. 12).

Irregular narrow-complex tachycardias

- Atrial fibrillation with an uncontrolled ventricular response (Fig. 13).

- Atrial flutter with irregular AV conduction (variable block and hence irregular).

Other investigations

- Electrolytes: hypokalaemia, hypomagnesaemia and acidosis can precipitate arrhythmias.

- FBC: anaemia will exacerbate myocardial ischaemia.

- CXR: heart size and pulmonary oedema.

- Echocardiogram: left ventricular function and other anatomical abnormality.

Management

Tachycardia causing haemodynamic compromise in an unstable patient

Synchronised DC cardioversion is required: the energy levels will depend on the underlying rhythm, the type of defibrillator (biphasic or monophasic) and whether the patient is on digoxin.

- Atrial flutter/SVT: 25 J (monophasic).

- Atrial fibrillation: 100 J.

- Ventricular tachycardia: 100 J.

If cardioversion is unsuccessful, try moving the paddles to the anterior/posterior position with one paddle over the heart apex and the other below the right scapula to the right of the spine.

Tachycardia not causing haemodynamic compromise

Management will depend on the cause.

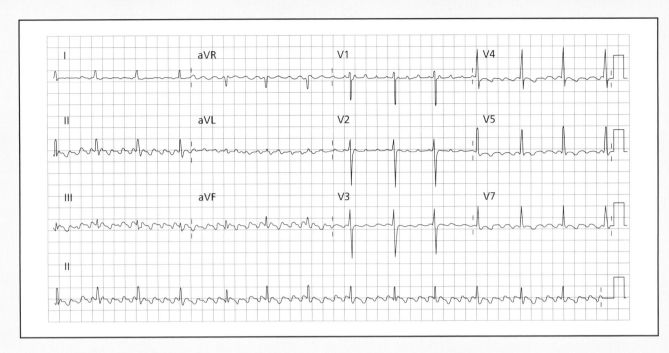

▲**Fig. 12** Atrial flutter with 4:1 AV block.

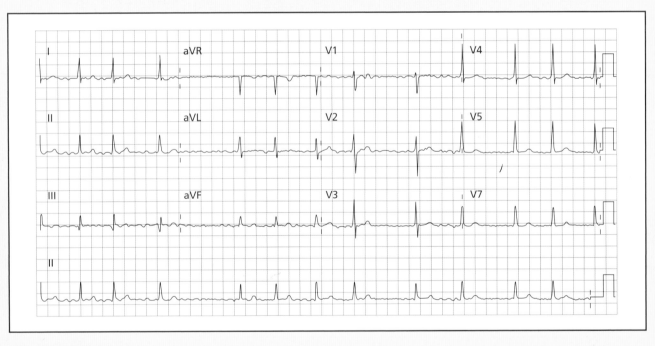

▲**Fig. 13** Atrial fibrillation.

Sinus tachycardia Management should be directed at the underlying cause: attempts to slow the arrhythmia by any other means will almost certainly do more harm than good.

Supraventricular tachycardia Vagal manoeuvres or adenosine are the treatments of choice. Vagal manoeuvres (Valsalva and carotid sinus massage, etc.) should be used with caution and only by those with experience.

Adenosine is a naturally occurring purine nucleoside that is highly efficient at blocking the AV node. Its action lasts for seconds only, and it is not negatively inotropic. It is highly effective at terminating paroxysmal SVT with re-entrant circuits that include the AV node (AV re-entrant tachycardia and AV nodal re-entrant tachycardia). In other narrow-complex tachycardias (eg atrial flutter) it will reveal the underlying atrial rhythm by slowing the ventricular response.

Adenosine should be administered as follows:

- start with a rapid intravenous bolus of 6 mg;
- follow with up to two doses of 12 mg at intervals of 1–2 minutes;
- each bolus should be followed immediately by a flush of saline into a large vein.

Adenosine is contraindicated in the following patients:

- those with asthma;
- those with high-degree AV block (second- or third-degree heart block);
- those taking dipyridamole (potentiates the effect of adenosine).

If adenosine is contraindicated or fails to terminate a regular narrow-complex tachycardia without demonstrating that it is atrial flutter, then give a calcium channel blocker (verapamil or diltiazem). Beta-blockers are a reasonable alternative.

Irregular broad-complex tachycardia Be cautious in the management of an irregular broad-complex tachycardia. If it is atrial fibrillation with bundle branch block, treat as for atrial fibrillation (see below). If pre-excitation is present, then adenosine, digoxin and verapamil should be avoided; these drugs block the AV node and may increase accessory pathway conduction with the inherent danger of precipitating ventricular fibrillation.

Atrial fibrillation Many patients with atrial fibrillation of recent onset will eventually cardiovert to sinus rhythm irrespective of the treatment strategy used. These patients are at risk of stroke and antithrombotic therapy takes priority over the

treatment of rate or rhythm, although in each individual patient both the risks and benefits of anticoagulation need to be carefully considered.

In haemodynamically stable patients where atrial fibrillation is known to be of recent onset (<48 hours) and not precipitated by intercurrent illness, the patient should undergo electrical cardioversion. If that fails, pharmacological cardioversion should be attempted. Amiodarone is both antiarrhythmic and rate limiting (see below for dosing regimen). Alternatives include digoxin (orally, loading regimen 1.0–1.5 mg in divided doses over 24 hours), particularly in the presence of left ventricular dysfunction, and beta-blockers. Long-term antithrombotic treatment is not required if a patient is thought to be at low risk of recurrence of atrial fibrillation after restoration of sinus rhythm.

If atrial fibrillation has been present for longer than 48 hours and was not precipitated by intercurrent illness the priority, after antithrombotic treatment, is rate control with beta-blockers or digoxin. Elective cardioversion at 6 weeks can be considered.

If a patient in atrial fibrillation has WPW syndrome, then AV node blocking drugs (including digoxin) should be avoided. Flecainide is an alternative, but not in the presence of left ventricular dysfunction. Call for specialist advice rather than 'having a go'.

If a patient is known to be in permanent atrial fibrillation and the ventricular rate is poorly controlled, a rate-control strategy should be used. Options include beta-blockers or a rate-limiting calcium antagonist: where these are

ineffective or contraindicated, amiodarone remains an option.

Regular broad-complex tachycardia
In the absence of adverse features, give amiodarone 300 mg iv over 20–60 minutes followed by 900 mg in the next 24 hours. Procainamide and sotalol are reasonable alternatives. Class 1c drugs should be avoided. Monitor the patient closely. If adverse features develop, be prepared to use electrical cardioversion. If the arrhythmia persists, the patient should be referred for consideration of an implantable cardioverter defibrillator. Intravenous magnesium should be used for patients with polymorphic VT.

An algorithm to help in the diagnosis of broad-complex tachycardia is shown in Fig. 14.

In the haemodynamically stable patient, give one antiarrhythmic agent. If this is unsuccessful in restoring normal rhythm, it will be safer to move to DC cardioversion rather than administering additional antiarrhythmic drugs.

1.2.7 Bradyarrhythmia

Scenario

A 76-year-old woman is brought to the Emergency Department by ambulance having been found collapsed in her kitchen at home by her son when he went round to visit in the morning. She is normally independent and lives alone. She has a past medical history of hypertension, osteoarthritis and non-insulin-dependent diabetes mellitus. You are called to review her urgently by the triage nurse, who finds her pulse rate to be 30 bpm.

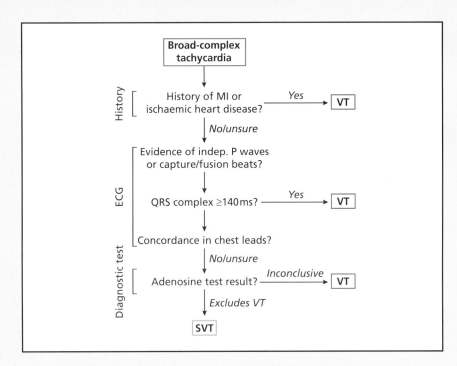

▲**Fig. 14** Algorithm to help decision-making in broad-complex tachycardia. MI, myocardial infarction; SVT, supraventricular tachycardia; VT, ventricular tachycardia.

Introduction

The first priority will be to check her other vital signs and make a judgement as to whether she is well enough to give a useful history. She may be tolerating her bradycardia well and be able to give an account of what has happened to her, but if she is not then you should immediately proceed from a rapid screening examination (head-to-toe screen and Glasgow Coma Scale/Abbreviated Mental Test Score, as appropriate) to treatment.

The most obvious diagnosis from the details given is that the woman has developed complete heart block, but do not jump to conclusions: if she had a simple trip in the evening but hurt herself such that she could not get off the floor, then she may have a bradycardia due to hypothermia in the morning.

History of the presenting problem

If the patient is well enough to give a history, then pursue an account of the collapse itself. What details (if any) can she (or her son) remember? Try to get a precise account: 'What exactly were you doing? Then what happened . . . and then?' Note in particular the following.

- Did she get any warning? Absence of warning symptoms would be typical of cardiac syncope (Stokes–Adams attack).

- How long did it last? In most cases of cardiac syncope the period of unconsciousness usually lasts 10–30 seconds.

- Did she injure herself when she collapsed?

- How did the son find her? Is there any evidence that she may have spent the night on the floor? Was she fully clothed when found, and what was the ambient temperature of her surroundings? If she spent the night on the floor, then it means that following the collapse she was not able to mobilise sufficiently to call for help or return to bed, which may

have important implications in relation to the cause of the collapse. Also, spending the night on the floor will increase her risk of developing hypothermia, pressure sores and other associated injuries.

Other relevant history

Has she had previous similar events: syncope or presyncope? Is there any history of epilepsy or any features to suggest that she could have had an unwitnessed fit (although this does not seem likely in this case)?

What medication is she on and have any drugs been started recently? Enquire specifically about antihypertensives (especially beta-blockers), but also hypoglycaemic agents, analgesics, sedatives and antiparkinsonian medications, all of which can cause confusion and/or disturbance of consciousness.

Examination

If the woman is very unwell proceed as described in Section 1.2.2, but otherwise concentrate on the following.

- What is she wearing? This may have some relevance as to at what time the collapse occurred.

- Signs of injury: in particular look at the pressure areas for signs that she has been immobile for a period. Specifically consider whether she has a fractured hip by looking for a short, externally rotated leg.

- Temperature: is she hypothermic? Use a low-reading thermometer and take a rectal temperature.

- Cardiovascular: check heart rate and rhythm, peripheral perfusion and BP. Automated machines may give unreliable results in a patient with low cardiac output due to bradycardia, so check a manual BP reading.

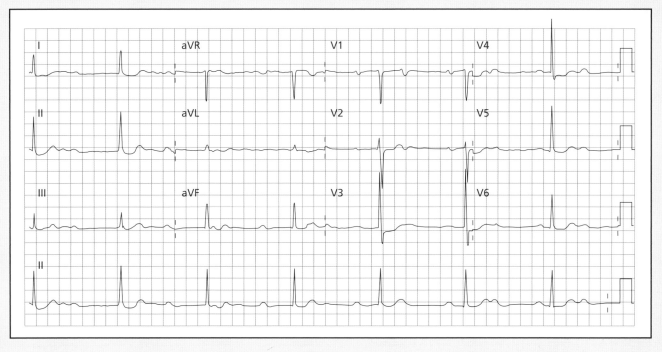

▲**Fig. 15** Complete heart block with a ventricular rate of 41/minute: whether immediate pacing is required will depend on the clinical context.

- Respiratory: are there signs to suggest aspiration/hypostatic pneumonia?

- Neurological: assess using the Glasgow Coma Scale; also look for focal signs that might indicate she has had a stroke (most commonly dysphasia, hemianopia, facial asymmetry and hemiparesis).

- Signs to suggest hypothyroidism: general appearance and slow-relaxing tendon jerks.

> ⚠ Do not forget hypothermia as a cause of profound bradycardia, especially in the elderly.

Investigation

ECG
Is there heart block (Fig. 15) and, if so, is it first-, second- or third-degree in type? Generally speaking, the higher the degree of heart block, the less stable the situation. But this is by no means always the case and the decision on management should not be taken on the basis of the ECG alone. Alternatively, there may be atrial fibrillation with a slow ventricular response or even profound sinus bradycardia. Is there any indication of recent myocardial infarction (MI) that might demand specific treatment?

Routine blood tests
Electrolytes, renal/liver/bone profile, glucose, creatine kinase (CK), troponin I/T and thyroid function tests. A very high CK (>10,000 IU/L) with hypocalcaemia and hyperphosphataemia is typically seen with rhabdomyolysis. A grossly elevated troponin would indicate MI, but a lesser elevation would be non-specific. Similarly a grossly elevated thyroid-stimulating hormone level (>20 IU/L) would indicate hypothyroidism, but a more modest increase would not be interpretable.

Urine
Dipstick for blood and protein. If positive for blood, check microscopy for red cells. A positive dipstick with no red cells is caused by urinary myoglobin in rhabdomyolysis.

Other tests
- CXR.

- CT scan of the brain.

- Blood (and other) cultures depending on clinical suspicion.

- Arterial blood gases if patient very unwell.

Management
Any clear cause of bradycardia or complication of the collapse should be treated on its merits. However, if the diagnosis is simply 'heart block' with no obvious precipitant that can be removed, then management should depend on the state of the patient:

If the patient is well
Some patients can tolerate complete heart block at a pulse rate of 30 bpm if their left ventricular function is good. They may be fully conscious

with a normal BP and warm peripheries. If this is the case, immediate transvenous pacing is not necessary and an elective decision on the need for a permanent pacing system can be taken. Close observation and cardiac monitoring is mandatory.

> If a patient is tolerating the bradycardia, then temporary transvenous pacing is almost certainly not needed.

If the patient is unwell

Immediate temporary cardiac pacing may be required if the patient is symptomatic. Marked bradyarrhythmia in someone who has suffered loss of consciousness, albeit transient, is almost certainly an indication for cardiac pacing, and the decision between a temporary transvenous procedure or the emergency insertion of a permanent system depends on local resources. Heart block with normal, narrow QRS complexes (<120 ms), as shown in Fig. 15, suggests a nodal source of ventricular depolarisation and is less likely to require an immediate temporary pacemaker. Other treatments that may be helpful include the following.

- Atropine (initial dose 0.5–1 mg iv): this may speed up the patient's ventricular rate and buy time while temporary pacing is organised.

- Isoprenaline (infusion rate 2–10 µg/min iv, with a drug half-life of approximately 2 minutes): may be useful *in extremis.*

- External cardiac pacemaker: may be used while arrangements are made for a definitive procedure.

Further comments

Bradycardia and myocardial infarction

The combination of acute MI and bradyarrhythmia requiring temporary pacing presents a challenge. The procedure carries extra risk following thrombolysis. Insert the pacing wire through the femoral vein so that pressure can be applied if there is bleeding, although this is impossible in the neck (the brachial is an alternative route, but manoeuvring the tip of the wire is often very difficult). If a wire has already been inserted through the internal jugular or subclavian vein in the context of acute MI, most would then advocate that thrombolysis should not be undertaken.

Hypothermia

A core body temperature of less than 33°C is diagnostic of hypothermia (Fig. 16). The management principles differ according to the cause of the lowered temperature.

- Rapid onset: in young patients the lowering of body temperature is often rapid, eg after immersion in water or collapse on a cold city street following alcohol intoxication. Rapid ('active', 'intensive') warming is required.

- Gradual onset: in most cases of hypothermia in the elderly the fall in body temperature occurs over several days, and so warming should be more gentle (warm bedding and a space blanket). Indeed there is some evidence that intensive warming in the elderly causes cardiovascular collapse and arrhythmias.

Broad-spectrum antibiotics should be given empirically: pneumonia (both hypostatic and aspiration) is a complicating feature of abnormally low body temperature.

Hypothyroidism

Hypothyroidism is associated with a variety of bradyarrhythmias, particularly sinus bradycardia and atrial fibrillation with a slow ventricular rate. In acute severe hypothyroidism, steroids should be given before starting thyroid replacement; without them, thyroid replacement therapy can result in acute circulatory collapse. Elderly patients often have coexisting ischaemic heart disease and their hypothyroidism will have developed over a considerable period of time. Vigorous replacement of thyroid hormone may well do more harm than good, hence the starting dose of thyroxine should be very small, 25 µg daily, or administered on alternate days. Triiodothyronine is rarely indicated.

Overdose with beta-blockers

Glucagon acts to reverse the effects of cardiovascular depression assosiated with beta-blocker overdose. The initial dosage is 5 mg, repeated as necessary. It may be necessary to start an infusion of glucagon if a long-acting beta-blocker has been taken.

1.2.8 Collapse of unknown cause

Scenario

A 70-year-old man has been brought to the Emergency Department. He was found by his daughter on the kitchen floor. He has poor recollection of events and his daughter did not see what happened. He has a history of Parkinson's disease and mild dementia. From the end of the bed you can see that he has a cut to the back of his head and one on his left forearm. What caused the collapse?

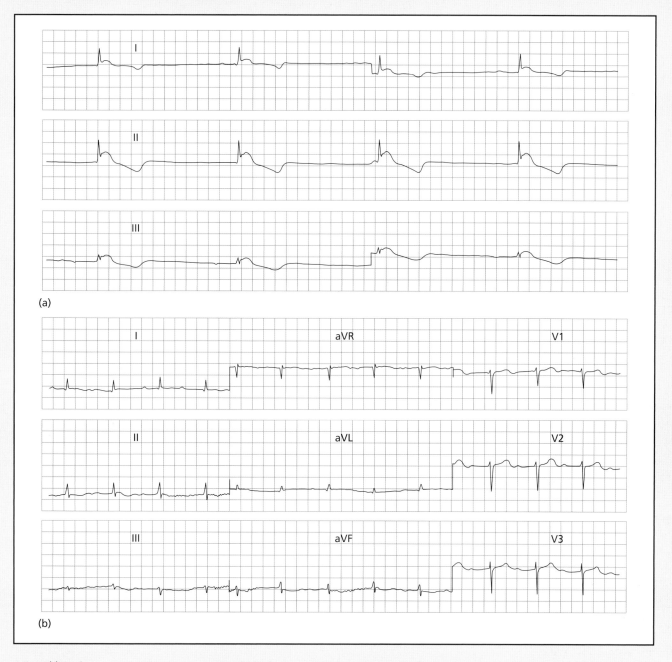

▲ **Fig. 16 (a)** ECG from a patient with a core temperature of 25°C, showing profound sinus bradycardia, first-degree heart block and prominent 'J' waves. **(b)** ECG from the same patient after warming to 31°C, showing heart rate 75 bpm, persistent first-degree heart block and no 'J' waves.

Introduction

'Collapse of unknown cause' is one of the commonest and yet one of the most difficult differential diagnoses in acute medicine. The case described here is typical: an elderly person has fallen to the floor, perhaps injuring themselves in the process, and sorting out what has happened and why is problematic

because (i) the patient is often unable to give a clear account, (ii) there is a wide differential diagnosis of syncope (Table 2) and (iii) the 'collapse' may not have a single cause – the blame may be attributable to the combination of a loose carpet, poor vision, an arthritic knee and recent introduction of antihypertensive therapy.

History of the presenting problem

Consider the conditions listed in Table 2 as you take the history, looking in particular for the following clues.

Neurally mediated syncope

Patients with vasovagal syncope will typically give a long history of syncope, which occurs after sudden,

TABLE 2 CAUSES OF SYNCOPE

Type of cause	Common example	Less common or rare example

Neurologically mediated	Vasovagal syncope
	Postural (orthostatic) hypotension
	Situational syncope
	  Urinating (micturition syncope)
	  Coughing (cough syncope)
	Carotid sinus syncope
		Situational syncope
		  Defecating (defecation syncope)
		  Swallowing (deglutition syncope)
		  Post-exercise/postprandial syncope
		Autonomic failure
		  Parkinson's disease (some patients)
		  Diabetic neuropathy
		Cerebrovascular, eg subclavian steal syndrome

Cardiac	Cardiac arrhythmia Aortic stenosis	Pulmonary artery hypertension Atrial myxoma
Neurological	Epilepsy	Hypoglycaemia

suggestive of a complex partial seizure. Tongue biting and urinary incontinence clearly support the diagnosis of epilepsy, but note that the presence of jerking limbs and incontinence do not conclusively establish epilepsy as the primary cause. Anoxic fits can occur following prolonged cerebral anoxia, such as when a patient remains propped up after passing out.

! Jerking limbs and urinary incontinence do not prove that epilepsy is the primary cause of a collapse.

unexpected and unpleasant sights, sounds, smells or pain, or after prolonged standing or sitting in crowded hot places. The syncope may occur during a meal or in the absorptive state after a meal. Typical prodromal symptoms include light-headedness, ringing in the ears, visual disturbances, sweating and/or nausea/vomiting. Vasovagal syncope is uncommon after early adulthood (so be very reluctant to make this diagnosis in this case). In the much rarer condition of carotid sinus syncope, head rotation puts pressure on the carotid sinus and leads to syncope.

Orthostatic hypotension

This typically occurs soon after standing up, but also on prolonged standing, especially in crowded hot places. Look for a temporal relationship between presentation and the start or change in dosage of any antihypertensives and Parkinson's disease treatments (levodopa and dopamine agonists) in particular. Orthostatic hypotension frequently occurs in patients with autonomic neuropathy or parkinsonism.

Cardiac syncope

Syncope associated with effort, chest pain, shortness of breath or palpitations is more likely to have a cardiac cause (see *Cardiology*, Section 1.4.1). These can occur when supine. A witness account of pallor followed by flushing would be very suggestive of a Stokes–Adams attack (due to the intermittent development of complete heart block) but does not occur in all patients with this condition (see *Cardiology*, Sections 1.4.1 and 2.2.1). Cardiac syncope is more likely in the presence of definite structural heart disease, and be aware of those with a family history of sudden death.

Excluding cardiac syncope as the cause of collapse is important as these patients have a higher mortality than those with non-cardiac causes.

Epilepsy

If the patient was awake during an attack, ask specifically about any warnings that he or any witness may have noticed. Features such as lip smacking, fiddling with clothes or stereotyped movements would be

It will clearly also be important to get a more detailed history of the patient's other medical conditions and of the wider social picture: organising appropriate discharge and placement for a man with mild dementia and Parkinson's disease who has fallen at home may not be straightforward.

Examination

Aside from establishing that there are no injuries from the fall following the collapse, particularly look for a short externally rotated leg from a fractured neck of femur or for injury to the neck. Then look for the following.

- Heart rate, rhythm and character.

- Postural BP: orthostatic BP measurements are recommended after 5 minutes of lying supine, followed by measurements each minute, or more often, while standing for 3 minutes. If the patient does not tolerate standing for this period, the lowest systolic BP during the upright posture should be recorded. A decrease in systolic BP ≥20 mmHg or a decrease in the level of systolic

BP to <90 mmHg is defined as orthostatic hypotension regardless of whether or not symptoms occur.

- Does the patient have a pacemaker?

- Heart murmur: in particular of aortic stenosis.

- Peripheral pulses: including auscultation of carotid arteries.

- Neurological: any focal signs, most likely attributable to stroke in this context, but also conceivably due to subdural haemorrhage in this patient who has banged his head.

Investigation
Immediate investigations would be as described in Section 1.2.7, with other radiological studies as dictated by clinical suspicion (X-ray of arm or hip?). Additional consideration should be given to:

- 24-hour ambulatory ECG, which will be required if cardiac syncope is suspected (it will not be evident on the resting ECG);

- postural testing on a tilt table.

Management
Management will depend on the precise diagnosis.

- Education: to avoid trigger events, recognise the onset symptoms and teach manoeuvres to abort episodes.

- Postural hypotension: requires a review of current medication and consideration of treatment with fludrocortisone or midodrine.

- Cardiac arrhythmia: may require permanent pacemakers/ defibrillators and/or drug therapy.

- Seizures: a convincing history warrants treatment with

antiepileptics, but these should not be given as a therapeutic trial when the clinical picture is not compelling.

1.2.9 Asthma

Scenario

A 36-year-old woman who has had asthma since childhood is admitted with progressive breathlessness and cough. You are asked to assess her: is the attack serious? Does she need to be admitted or could she go home with treatment?

History of the presenting problem
The following questions are important in assessing the severity of, and appropriate response to, this attack.

- How long has she been breathless? The duration of the illness may be short and her deterioration rapid; equally there may be a history of illness for a few days prior to admission in association with progressive breathlessness. Both sets of circumstances may be equally severe, but you would want to monitor much more closely the patient who seemed to be getting worse rapidly.

- Has she had variation in severity during the day or at night? Diurnal variation and nocturnal symptoms are important pointers to deterioration in asthmatics. Progressive and nocturnal symptoms probably indicate a loss of control of disease prior to presentation. If background control has been poor, recovery following treatment is often delayed.

- Has she been using more of her normal medication? If so, has it

helped? Most asthmatics are used to their disease and will try to avoid coming to hospital. To avoid admission they often self-medicate with increasing amounts up to the point at which it is not helping.

- Although the presumption is that the problem is due to an attack of asthma, are there any features that are unusual? Has she been feverish, suggesting a precipitating infection? Has she had pleuritic chest pain that may indicate a spontaneous pneumothorax?

Other relevant history
It will be important to establish how well/poorly controlled her asthma usually is, and whether or not she monitors it.

- How debilitating is her asthma normally and what can't she do because of it? Does she ever measure her peak flow and, if so, what are the readings?

- How frequently does she have attacks of asthma and how bad have they been? How many times has she needed to see her GP or to be admitted to hospital in the last 12 months? When was her last course of steroids? Has she ever needed to be admitted to a high-dependency unit (HDU) or an intensive care unit (ICU), and has she ever needed artificial ventilation? These are always worrying features.

- What medication does she take normally? The need for home nebulisers and/or maintenance steroids probably signifies poorly controlled or 'brittle' asthma. In addition to any medication she may be taking for her asthma, it is important to ask whether she is on any other new medications or if she has recently received antibiotics or steroids in the community.

TABLE 3 BTS GUIDELINES (2003) FOR ASSESSING THE SEVERITY OF ACUTE ASTHMA

Severity	Features
Acute severe asthma	Peak expiratory flow rate (PEFR) 33–50% of best (use per cent predicted if best unknown) Cannot complete sentences in one breath Respiratory rate >25/minute Pulse >110 bpm
Life-threatening	PEFR <33% of best or predicted Sao_2 <92% Silent chest, cyanosis or feeble respiratory effort Bradycardia, arrhythmia or hypotension Exhaustion, confusion or coma
Near-fatal asthma	Raised $Paco_2$ Requires intermittent positive-pressure ventilation with raised inflation pressures

Examination

The British Thoracic Society (BTS) guidelines for assessing the severity of acute asthma are given in Table 3.

General

> When examining this patient it is most important to check the following.
>
> - Does she look dead or nearly dead? Get help quickly.
> - Does she appear agitated or exhausted? Get help quickly.
> - Can she speak in full sentences, only in words or is she unable to speak? If only in words or unable to speak, get help quickly.
> - Is she cyanosed? If she is, she is nearly dead.

Respiratory

It is important to measure respiratory rate, but the degree of tachypnoea does not correlate with the severity of an asthma attack. Asthma is a terrifying condition and most acute asthmatics hyperventilate, but then their respiratory rate falls as they become exhausted with the effort of breathing, eventually leading to hypercapnic respiratory failure and the need for ventilatory support.

> Respiratory rate must be interpreted in the context of the whole patient: a normal respiratory rate is consistent with imminent death in the asthmatic who is becoming exhausted.

Widespread wheezing indicates airways obstruction, but beware the asthmatic who has a silent chest on auscultation: the tidal volume may be reduced so much that insufficient flow is being generated to create a wheeze. Check for signs of an underlying pneumothorax and for pneumonic consolidation.

Cardiovascular

Sinus tachycardia is common in acute asthma and does not correlate with severity. Fear, increased sympathetic drive and bronchodilator drugs all contribute to a rise in pulse rate. Bradycardia may supervene as hypoxia becomes more marked.

The degree of pulsus paradoxus (exaggeration of the normal fall in systolic BP on inspiration) does correlate with severity of asthma as it reflects the abnormal changes in transpulmonary pressure generated by increasing airways obstruction.

> No clinical sign correlates well with the degree of hypoxia: measure arterial blood gases at the earliest opportunity!

Investigation

- Peak flow: is she too tired to attempt this? How does the value now compare with her usual one and how do you interpret the result? (See Table 3.)

- Pulse oximetry: will be useful in detection of hypoxia, but the absence of hypoxia does not guarantee that all is well.

> Oximetry only gives part of the picture: it quantifies arterial oxygenation but does not tell you how well a patient is ventilating. A patient given high-flow oxygen might not be hypoxic but could still be hypoventilating and be at risk of respiratory arrest.

- Arterial blood gases: mandatory in all but the mildest cases. Initially you may see slight hypoxia/normoxia with reduced $Paco_2$, suggesting hyperventilation in order to maintain adequate oxygenation. Hypoxia, hypercapnia and acidosis ensue as the patient tires. A metabolic acidosis in acute asthma is a bad prognostic sign, suggesting impaired cardiac output due to severe airflow obstruction.

Most patients with asthma hate having arterial blood gases taken due to previous bad experiences. A 22G needle is perfectly adequate, rather than a 20G or even an 18G. If local anaesthetic is required, warm it up to reduce the stinging.

- CXR: look carefully and deliberately for a pneumothorax, consolidation due to superadded infection or segmental collapse due to sputum plugging.

- Routine blood investigations: FBC (anaemia will compound impaired tissue oxygen delivery) and electrolytes (β_2-agonists, theophyllines and steroids all predispose to hypokalaemia, which can create a respiratory myopathy).

- ECG: sinus tachycardia will be the likely finding, but it is important to exclude any tachyarrhythmias that may result primarily as a result of cardiac compromise or secondarily to treatment strategies (ie β_2-agonists or theophyllines).

Management

Assuming that the history and examination are consistent with the diagnosis of an acute exacerbation of asthma, then oxygen, bronchodilators and steroids are the first-line treatments.

- Oxygen: maximum inspired oxygen by face mask should be administered. This is best achieved by using a mask with a reservoir bag that can deliver inspired oxygen concentrations of 85% at a flow rate of 15 L/min. Do not be concerned about high-flow oxygen in this situation: it will not cause progressive hypoventilation and hypercapnia, although these might occur if the patient becomes exhausted.

- Bronchodilators: combining anticholinergic drugs with β_2-agonists confers additional benefit in acute asthma. Nebulised therapy should be given early and repeated frequently in the early stages of an acute attack: salbutamol (5–10 mg) can be nebulised with ipratropium (500 µg) and repeated as necessary.

 Ensure that the nebuliser is driven by oxygen and not air!

- Steroids: give prednisolone 40–50 mg orally if the patient is able to take it. There is no evidence that intravenous hydrocortisone confers additional benefit in acute asthma. Current guidelines recommend concurrent administration of oral and intravenous preparations if patients are very ill and compliant with both forms of therapy.

What do you do if the patient does not improve?

It is vital that senior clinician support and ICU support is requested sooner rather than later. Do not delay: asthmatics can deteriorate rapidly.

If life-threatening features are present or the patient does not improve with the initial treatment after 15–30 minutes, then further treatments needs to be administered.

- Intravenous magnesium sulphate 1.2–2.0 g over 20 minutes. This works as a calcium antagonist that induces smooth muscle relaxation. A single dose of intravenous magnesium sulphate has been shown to be effective and safe in acute severe asthma (the safety of repeated doses is yet to be assessed).

- Intravenous bronchodilators: aminophylline should be used with caution, especially if oral theophyllines are part of the patient's regular medication. The potential complications of aminophylline toxicity (epileptic convulsions and/or vomiting) are extremely dangerous in acute asthma. Salbutamol can be used as an alternative and is preferred by many: dilute 5 mg in 500 mL of 5% dextrose or 0.9% saline and start infusion at a rate of 7.5 µg/min, titrating according to response. The main side effects are tachycardia and tremor.

The β_2-agonists and aminophylline must always be given with oxygen, not instead of it. These drugs are pulmonary vasodilators as well as bronchodilators and their administration can rapidly worsen ventilation–perfusion mismatch, causing a reduction in Pao_2 unless supplemental oxygen is given.

- Intravenous fluids: hyperventilation and poor oral intake can lead to dehydration. Dry bronchial secretions are more difficult to clear and can lead to sputum plugging. A relatively high right ventricular filling pressure is necessary in patients with severe airways obstruction to safeguard cardiac output. Do not be frightened to give 1 L of crystalloid in the first 1–2 hours.

Regular clinical reassessment of the patient is crucial, supplemented by repeated measurement of PEFR 15–30 minutes after commencing treatment, oximetry and arterial blood gas measurements.

Further comments

Patients with asthma still die. It is important to remember that early review by the ICU is important. If the patient is admitted *in extremis* or does not improve with treatment, get help. The move to the ICU should be a cool elective decision, not a panic when the patient is close to respiratory arrest. Important pointers to a deterioration may include:

- previous admission to an ICU/HDU;

- exhaustion, feeble respirations, confusion or drowsiness;

- deteriorating PEFR;

- worsening or persisting hypoxia or hypercapnia.

1.2.10 Pleurisy

Scenario

A 22-year-old woman is referred to the Emergency Department because of the sudden onset of right-sided pleuritic chest pain. She has no previous medical or surgical history. She has taken oral contraception for the past 12 months. Her GP writes 'I would be grateful if you could exclude a pulmonary embolus as the cause of her symptoms'.

Introduction

This is a pulmonary embolism (PE) until proved otherwise. Priorities are as follows.

- Airway, breathing and circulation (ABC).

- Is the patient ill? If so, administer high-flow oxygen and monitor pulse oximetry; check respiratory rate, heart rate and BP; obtain intravenous access; and give fluid bolus if hypotensive. Cardiovascular collapse indicates massive PE and is an indication for thrombolysis: call for senior help earlier rather than later.

- Low-molecular-weight heparin: this should be administered without delay to protect against further embolisation in all patients with a high probablity of PE. Doctors often delay giving heparin until they have completed taking the history, examined the patient and obtained the result of initial investigations.

- Analgesia: pleurisy is painful! Relieve the pain as soon as possible. NSAIDs are excellent for relieving the pain of pleurisy, but opiates may be required as well.

> If it is clear that PE is the number one diagnosis, start treatment immediately unless there are obvious pressing contraindications.

History of the presenting problem

Look specifically for features in the history that would point to a diagnosis of PE.

- Pain: did it start suddenly or gradually? The former is typical of PE, but a gradual onset of symptoms does not exclude the diagnosis. Sudden onset of pain (and/or breathlessness) after defecation is highly suggestive of PE, and there is commonly a story of becoming suddenly very frightened (a sense of impending doom).

- Breathlessness: post-mortem studies show that patients who die of PE virtually always have evidence that embolisms have occurred over a period of time. Has she had recent breathlessness or had to slow down?

- Haemoptysis: the commonest differential diagnosis of pleurisy is musculoskeletal pain, and this does not cause haemoptysis.

- Calf/leg swelling or pain: these would suggest deep venous thrombosis (DVT) and strongly support the diagnosis of PE in this clinical context.

- Has the patient had a DVT or PE before?

- Is there a major risk factor? Ask about recent immobility/major surgery/lower limb trauma or surgery, pregnancy/postpartum, any major medical illness, taking oral contraceptives (as in this case) and a family history of such illnesses.

> **Pitfalls in the diagnosis of PE**
>
> Pleuritic pain is not always a feature of PE: large central emboli typically cause cardiovascular collapse and breathlessness; smaller, more peripheral emboli tend to cause pain.

> **Differential diagnosis of pleurisy**
>
> - Spontaneous pneumothorax: heparin can convert this into a haemothorax.
> - Pneumonia: fever is often a prominent symptom, and chest signs and radiography will usually show consolidation. However, fever and radiographic consolidation can be a feature of pulmonary infarction.
> - Musculoskeletal pain: this can be difficult to differentiate. If the diagnosis is unclear, anticoagulate until PE is excluded.
> - Less common and rare conditions: pain indistinguishable from pleurisy

can be due to shingles (herpes zoster) and pleurisy can be the presenting symptom of systemic lupus erythematosus, in which case check the relevant serology (antinuclear factor and DNA binding) and be particularly suspicious if pleurisy is recurrent.

Also remember that the presenting history (and findings) in PE may be dominated by secondary cardiac features, namely ischaemic cardiac pain and ECG changes. A PE creates a sudden increase in afterload on the right ventricle, and 'secondary cardiac pain' from the resulting myocardial ischaemia may be a prominent feature of the history.

Examination

The first priority will clearly be to make an assessment of the severity of illness (as described in Section 1.2.2). However, with regard to the particular diagnosis of PE, proceed as follows.

Cardiovascular

The most common sign is sinus tachycardia. BP may be elevated due to catecholamine release or may be reduced secondary to cardiovascular collapse. Most importantly, look for signs of pulmonary hypertension:

- elevated venous pressure, particularly with an exaggerated *a* wave;

- right ventricular heave, which can develop surprisingly rapidly following an acute rise in pulmonary artery pressure;

- right ventricular gallop rhythm and loud pulmonary second sound.

Respiratory

Most patients with a PE have a respiratory rate >20/minute, but

more specifically a pleural rub may be present. Always believe other medical staff if they describe a rub that is no longer present when you examine the patient.

 Chest wall tenderness

Patients with PE will tell you that it has been uncomfortable lying on the affected side and they may be locally tender on palpation. This is an important point because local tenderness does not necessarily mean pain of musculoskeletal origin: another classic diagnostic 'catch'.

Other features

Search for a DVT but do not be surprised if you do not find one. Also, do not let its absence put you off making the diagnosis of PE. A rectal examination (and pelvic examination in women) will be necessary at some stage, but not on admission of a patient who is breathless and unwell.

Investigation

Routine tests

All patients with this history require the following.

- CXR: in PE the findings are usually normal, but a number of radiographic abnormalities may occur, namely line shadows at the bases, peripheral wedge-shaped shadow(s), areas of relative oligaemia in the lung fields (rare) and enlarged proximal pulmonary artery (rare).

- ECG: in PE the ECG is commonly normal but it may show sinus tachycardia; T-wave inversion in V1–V3; an 'S1Q3T3' pattern, commonly described in the medical literature and reflecting axis change as a result of sudden increase in right ventricular

afterload (Fig. 17); right atrial hypertrophy with a 'P pulmonale'; right bundle branch block (can be a normal variant, but is significant if new); and evidence of ischaemic change, which may be left- or right-sided.

Other tests that may be appropriate include the following.

- D-dimer: only a negative result is of any value; hence it should only be measured where there is reasonable clinical suspicion of PE, but not where an alternative diagnosis is highly likely (when a 'positive' D-dimer will almost inevitably be a false positive) or if the clinical probability of PE is high (when the patient requires a definitive investigation, whatever the D-dimer result might be). In this case it would only be appropriate for you to measure D-dimer if you thought 'if this test is negative, I will reassure the woman, treat her symptomatically, and send her home'.

🔑 D-dimer is very helpful if used wisely, but it should not be used as a routine screening test for PE.

- Blood gases: these typically show hypocapnia in PE because of hyperventilation. Hypoxia may or may not be present. If there is a base deficit, your concerns should be heightened because it indicates secondary cardiovascular compromise. Calculation of the alveolar–arterial gradient may be helpful.

Definitive investigations

CT pulmonary angiography is now the imaging modality of choice (Fig. 18).

Ventilation–perfusion isotope lung scan may be considered as the initial

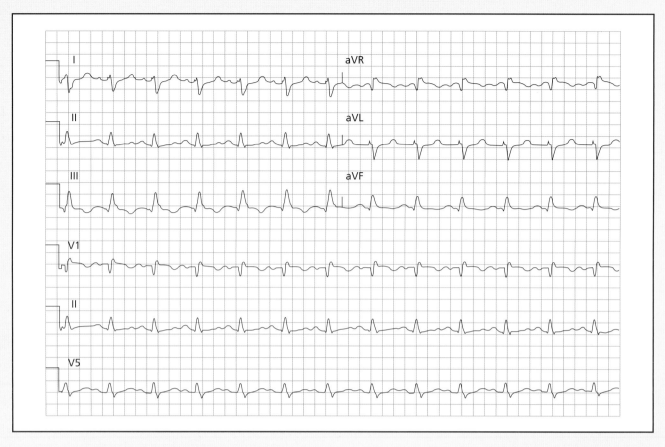

▲**Fig. 17** ECG in a case of acute PE showing the S1Q3T3 pattern.

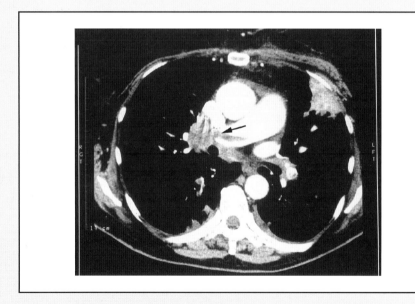

▲**Fig. 18** CT angiogram of the chest showing a clot in the proximal pulmonary artery (arrow).

Other tests

Routine haematological and biochemical tests should be performed: are there any clues to a systemic disease that might predispose to PE? A leg ultrasound scan is an alternative definitive imaging modality where there is clinical suspicion of a DVT, because identification of a DVT precludes the need for further tests. A patient with a proven DVT and pleuritic pain should be treated as if it is PE (because it is virtually impossible to think that the patient has not had one). There is a role for echocardiography in an unstable patient in whom the clinical suspicion of PE is high.

> ⚠ It is not possible to interpret the results of a thrombophilia screen in the presence of thrombus or anticoagulation.

imaging investigation provided the CXR is normal, there is no significant cardiopulmonary disease, standardised reporting criteria are used and a non-diagnostic result is always followed by further imaging. The presence of chronic lung or cardiac disease makes interpretation of ventilation–perfusion scans very difficult if not impossible (Fig. 19).

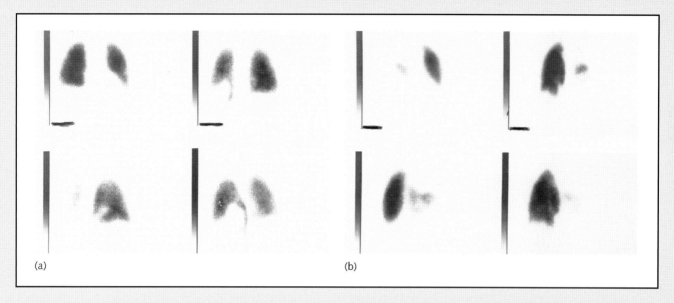

▲ **Fig. 19** Pulmonary emboli revealed on perfusion isotope lung scanning: (**a**) large segmental defect in the left lung; (**b**) virtually complete lack of perfusion in the right lung. Ventilation scanning was normal in both patients.

Management

Anticoagulation/thrombolysis

Low-molecular-weight heparin followed by warfarin will be appropriate for most patients, but occasionally thrombolytic agents will be indicated. There is no trial evidence to guide decision-making, but a common view would be that thrombolysis is indicated in patients with circulatory collapse or those who are persistently hypotensive from embolic disease despite heparin therapy. The current thrombolytic recommendation from the British Thoracic Society is for alteplase at the same dosage as that used in acute myocardial infarction.

Other aspects

If there is significant haemodynamic disturbance, then a high venous filling pressure is required to assist the struggling right ventricle. Give intravenous colloid (500 mL) swiftly and reassess. Close haemodynamic monitoring is required, ideally in the high-dependency unit or intensive care unit, so that deterioration can be spotted promptly and thrombolysis administered.

Repeated embolic events despite adequate anticoagulation may require mechanical intervention, eg insertion of a filter device into the inferior vena cava.

Important points to remember about PE

- Common and potentially life-threatening condition.
- Presentation is often atypical: if confronted with unexplained breathlessness or collapse, always consider the possibility of PE.
- Do not expect to find a predisposing cause for venous thrombosis.
- Examination is commonly unremarkable.
- CXR and ECG are commonly normal.
- CT angiography and ventilation–perfusion scans are particularly valuable soon after the clinical event: normal images obtained more than 48 hours after the clinical event do not exclude PE.
- Anticoagulate promptly while investigations are organised and the diagnosis is clarified. Give heparin. If the patient is very ill, do not hesitate to seek senior advice (the next PE may be fatal) and consider thrombolysis.

1.2.11 Chest infection/ pneumonia

Scenario

A 68-year-old woman with no significant past medical history is sent to the Medical Assessment Unit with a 48-hour history of fever, malaise, breathlessness and progressive confusion. The note from the referring GP suggests that she thinks the problem is pneumonia. You are asked to assess her.

History of the presenting problem

Pneumonia does seem the most likely diagnosis in this case, so pursue the symptoms described above and others that might be found in this condition.

- Fever: a low-grade fever is non-specific, but a fever of over 38.5°C in this context clearly supports pneumonia or another infective cause of illness (see Sections 1.2.33 and 1.2.34), as would the presence of rigors or 'chills'.

- Breathlessness: clearly supports the diagnosis of pneumonia, suggesting that there has been some ventilation–perfusion mismatch as may be seen with pneumonic consolidation.

- Cough: is there a cough and is it productive, purulent or dry? Does the woman normally have a cough and/or produce sputum? In the patient with normal lungs a dry cough is a common presenting feature of pneumonia of any sort; a purulent cough is indicative of an underlying bacterial infection; and brownish-red (rusty coloured) sputum is most likely due to pneumococcal infection.

- Chest pain: this may simply be due to 'sore ribs' from coughing or it may be pleuritic, which is more common in bacterial than non-bacterial infection.

- When did the illness start? The information given here suggests it was in the past 48 hours, but it is important to try to pinpoint the onset of symptoms or the prodromal stage of the illness. Non-bacterial causes of pneumonia (ie *Mycoplasma pneumoniae*) are often characterised by a relatively long prodromal stage in comparison with bacterial pneumonias.

- Confusion: indicates that the pneumonia is likely to be severe (see below), but note that the classic symptoms and signs of pneumonia are less likely in the elderly and so confusion may be the main presenting feature and only diagnostic clue.

- Is any other diagnosis more likely? Other common causes of acute presentation with breathlessness are pulmonary oedema or pulmonary embolism: are there features to support either of these

diagnoses? See Sections 1.2.5 and 1.2.10 for discussion. Remember that patients with atypical pneumonia commonly have gastrointestinal symptoms.

Other relevant history

A detailed past medical history is required, but issues of particular relevance include the following.

- Previous respiratory disease: does she have known chronic obstructive pulmonary disease, bronchiectasis or any other long-standing lung problems?

- Smoking history.

- Alcohol history: alcoholism may predispose the patient to aspiration as well as pneumococcal, Gram-negative and atypical infections. And it is important to recognise if a patient is likely to suffer from alcohol withdrawal if admitted to hospital.

- Pets: is there a parrot or budgie at home?

- Is she immunosuppressed?

Examination

A woman with pneumonia sufficient to cause confusion is likely to be very ill. Proceed as indicated in Section 1.2.2, but noting especially if there are signs of consolidation in the chest. A pleural rub is suggestive of bacterial pneumonia.

> ⚠ Remember that in non-bacterial pneumonia the respiratory signs are commonly unimpressive.

Investigation

Pulse oximetry/arterial blood gases

Oximetry is mandatory in all patients: those with Sao_2 <92% or features of severe pneumonia should

have arterial blood gas (ABG) measurements. A rising $Paco_2$ indicates failing ventilation and is a very worrying sign that should immediately trigger a request for senior support or input from the intensive care unit or both.

> ⚠ Measurement of oxygen saturation by pulse oximetry is likely to be inaccurate if there is poor peripheral perfusion, an instance when the early assessment of ABG is essential. Always document the inspired oxygen content when the ABG was taken.

Chest radiograph

Pneumococcal pneumonia presents classically as lobar or segmental consolidation (Fig. 20). Multiple, non-contiguous and sometimes bilateral segments may be affected, with multilobar involvement being a poor prognostic factor. The absence of an 'air bronchogram' within an area of consolidation suggests exudate or pus filling the conducting airways; aside from *Streptococcus pneumoniae*, organisms commonly responsible for this appearance include *Staphylococcus* (Fig. 21) and Gram-negative organisms. Early cavitation in an area of consolidation is typical of staphylococcal infection, but consider Gram-negative organisms such as *Klebsiella* and do not forget tuberculosis. Also consider aspiration pneumonia or proximal bronchial obstruction, eg due to carcinoma or a foreign body. A variety of radiographic patterns are described in *Mycoplasma* pneumonia (Fig. 22) and in Legionnaires' disease. The presence of pleural fluid is suggestive of bacterial aetiology and a diagnostic tap should be performed if this is anything more than trivial in size.

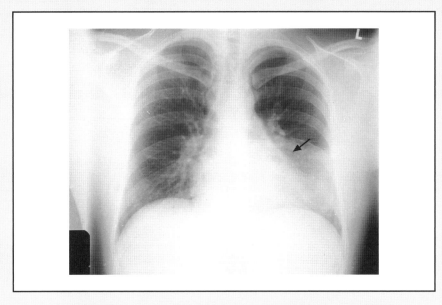

▲**Fig. 20** Lingular consolidation due to *Streptococcus pneumoniae*: the arrow marks an air bronchogram.

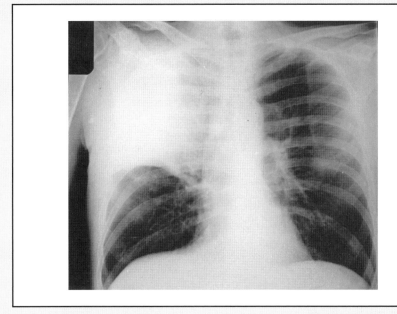

▲**Fig. 21** Dense consolidation with no air bronchogram due to staphylococcal pneumonia following influenza.

⚠ In pneumococcal pneumonia the radiograph may be normal at presentation, even in the presence of a classical history and signs of consolidation on examination, only to become abnormal over the next few hours.

Routine blood tests

Full blood count Anaemia will compound impaired tissue oxygen delivery and the white cell count is likely to be elevated. However, a patient with overwhelming sepsis may have a normal white cell count.

Electrolytes and renal function tests Uraemia is a bad prognostic sign in pneumonia (see CURB-65 below); hyponatraemia is another non-specific marker of the severity of illness, but is also (for unknown reasons) a particular feature of Legionnaires' disease.

Liver blood tests Derangement of liver enzymes may be seen in any severe sepsis, but note that transient hepatitis is seen as part of multisystem involvement in atypical infections (ie Legionnaires' disease). Also pay attention to inflammatory markers, ie C-reactive protein (CRP): a raised CRP on admission is a relatively more sensitive marker of pneumonia than an increased temperature or raised white cell count.

Microbiological tests

- Sputum microscopy and culture: if sputum is obtainable it is important to send a sample early in the illness; also do this for acid-fast bacilli if clinically indicated.

- Blood cultures.

- Urinary assays of specific antigens: pneumococcal antigen and *Legionella* antigen.

- Serological testing: send acute and convalescent titres for atypical serology.

- Pleural fluid, if there is significant effusion.

Management

General management and resuscitation (if required) should be as described in Sections 1.2.2 and 1.2.5, but note the following.

CURB-65 score

Assessment using CURB-65 (British Thoracic Society guidelines 2004) is vital as a prognostic indicator.

- Confusion: Mini-Mental State Examination <8, or new disorientation in person, place and time.
- Urea >7 mmol/L.
- Respiratory rate >30/minute.
- BP: systolic <90 mmHg or diastolic <60 mmHg.
- Age >65 years.

Score 1 point for each feature present; a score of 3–5 suggests severe pneumonia.

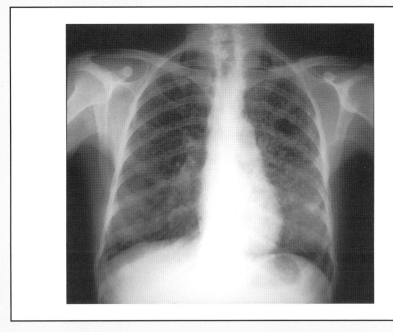

▲**Fig. 22** *Mycoplasma* pneumonia showing a lobular pattern of consolidation.

Antibiotics

Antibiotics should be given without delay, with the choice guided by the British Thoracic Society guidelines and/or local knowledge of the pathogens most commonly implicated. Always consult local prescribing policies in addition to obtaining microbiological advice as necessary.

- CURB-65 score 1 or 2: in the moderately sick patient, oral amoxicillin and a macrolide should be given. In those patients allergic to penicillin, a fluoroquinolone should be considered (ie levofloxacin).

- CURB-65 score 3 or more: in the more severely ill patient, co-amoxiclav or a third-generation cephalosporin should be given intravenously in conjunction with a macrolide. In patients who are penicillin allergic, an intravenous fluoroquinolone in addition to a macrolide should be considered.

- If Legionnaires' disease is suspected, then intravenous erythromycin 1 g every 6 hours should be included.

- If there is the suggestion of preceding influenza, consider adding a specific antistaphylococcal antibiotic, eg flucloxacillin.

- If Gram-negative infection or aspiration is suspected, then a third-generation cephalosporin is the antibiotic of choice.

Further comments

Remember that patients with severe pneumonia have high insensible losses due to hyperventilation and fever in addition to reduced oral intake: they may require up to 4 L/day of intravenous fluid, with careful clinical examination at least twice daily to ensure that they are not becoming volume depleted or overloaded.

Radiographic changes are not static and the radiograph may deteriorate during the early stages of treatment. However, if the radiograph deteriorates despite antibiotic therapy, you may not be covering the correct organism or the diagnosis of infection may be incorrect. Consider other pathologies, such as pulmonary infarction, pulmonary eosinophilia, cryptogenic organising pneumonia or pulmonary vasculitis (see *Respiratory Medicine*, Sections 2.7, 2.8.4 and 2.8.5).

1.2.12 Acute-on-chronic airways obstruction

Scenario

A 68-year-old man with a 50 pack-year history of smoking and known chronic obstructive pulmonary disease (COPD) has had increasing cough and breathlessness for the last 7 days and now presents to the Emergency Department. You are asked to assess him.

History of the presenting problem

You need to establish his normal level of respiratory function and the cause and severity of this deterioration.

Normal level of respiratory function and severity of deterioration

What is his usual exercise tolerance? How far can he normally walk? Can he climb a flight of stairs without stopping? How has his exercise capacity changed now? See the Medical Research Council dyspnoea scale below.

Medical Research Council dyspnoea scale

Grade of breathlessness is related to activities.

Grade 1   Not troubled by breathlessness, except on strenuous exercise.

Grade 2 Short of breath when hurrying or walking up a slight hill.

Grade 3 Walks slower than a contemporary on level ground because of breathlessness, or has to stop for breath when walking at own pace.

Grade 4 Stops for breath after walking about 100 m or after a few minutes on level ground.

Grade 5 Too breathless to leave the house, or breathless when dressing or undressing.

Cause of deterioration

The most likely explanation for deterioration is an acute exacerbation of COPD, but do not neglect to consider other possibilities. Important aspects of history to pursue include the following.

- What is his normal treatment and has this been increased recently? Ask particularly about steroids, recent courses of antibiotics, home nebulisers and home oxygen/ventilation.

- Fever and/or production of increasing amounts of purulent sputum, which would suggest an infective process.

- Chest pain: pleuritic pain could be due to pneumonia or fracture of a rib through coughing.

Could there be another diagnosis? Heavy smokers are clearly at risk of coronary heart disease and thereby left ventricular failure. How many pillows does the patient normally sleep with? Does he normally wake up at night due to breathlessness? Is this different from normal now? Do not over-interpret orthopnoea and paroxysmal nocturnal dyspnoea because any patient with respiratory difficulty will find it more difficult to breathe when lying down, but remember that left ventricular

failure and COPD commonly coexist. Are there any features to suggest pulmonary embolism (see Section 1.2.10)?

Other relevant history

A thorough past medical history is required, and also careful scrutiny of the patient's hospital notes (if available), with issues of particular relevance being the following.

- The number of admissions with respiratory problems in the past 5 years. Has high dependency care, intensive care or mechanical ventilation been required? This information is crucial if respiratory failure becomes inexorable and the appropriateness of assisted ventilation has to be decided.

- Social circumstances, including suitability of accommodation, will be important in considering discharge planning. Would this patient be suitable for the 'hospital at home/supported discharge' service available in many hospitals for patients with exacerbations of COPD?

Examination

As always, this should begin with an assessment of the overall severity of illness, as described in Section 1.2.2, with particular emphasis on two questions: what is the degree of respiratory distress and can pneumothorax be excluded? Hence look in particular for the following.

- Can the patient speak in sentences or just a few words at a time?

- Does he look exhausted?

- Is he using accessory muscles?

- Is he cyanosed?

- What is his respiratory rate? Remember, however, that a 'normal' respiratory rate is not a

reassuring finding in a patient who is becoming exhausted. An examination of the chest is likely to reveal scattered wheezes and crackles, but beware the silent chest and note if there is any consolidation suggesting pneumonia. Look in the sputum pot and check the peak expiratory flow rate.

Pneumothorax in chronic chest disease

Even a small pneumothorax can cause severe dyspnoea and distress in a person who has underlying chest disease.

Investigation

As in Section 1.2.11, but note the following.

- Arterial blood gases: prompt assessment is particularly important in this case because of the possibility that this patient might have type 2 respiratory failure with a high $P\text{co}_2$. A high $P\text{co}_2$ with a normal pH suggests chronic ventilatory failure, with an elevated bicarbonate level due to renal compensation (see *Respiratory Medicine*, Section 3.6.1).

- CXR: look specifically for a pneumothorax and/or focal lung pathology, which may be the result of infective consolidation or a bronchial carcinoma.

- Blood tests: aside from those detailed in Section 1.2.11, check the plasma level of theophyllines if the patient is taking these drugs.

Management

If the patient is *in extremis*, then resuscitation should proceed as described in Section 1.2.2.

> If a patient with known COPD looks very ill or worse, give high-flow oxygen to buy time for rapid assessment and instigation of ventilatory support. As stated before: hypoxia kills, hypercapnia merely intoxicates.

Management in a less severe case comprises the following.

- Oxygen: in patients who are not about to die, controlled oxygen (starting with 24%, given via a humidifier) is administered according to arterial blood gases, aiming to bring the Sao_2 above 92%. Arterial blood gases should be rechecked within 60 minutes of starting oxygen therapy and again within 60 minutes of a change in inspired oxygen. Humidification is important in order to decrease mucus plugging.

> Patients with asthma or COPD produce thick viscous secretions that significantly contribute to airway obstruction and are difficult to clear. Humidification of air/oxygen is simple, has no adverse side effects and helps greatly, so do not forget it.

- Bronchodilators: nebulised β_2-agonist (eg salbutamol 5 mg) and anticholinergic (eg ipratropium 500 µg), repeated as necessary.

- Steroids: start oral (eg prednisolone 30 mg od) or intravenous (eg hydrocortisone 200 mg qds) steroids.

- Antibiotics: amoxicillin 500 mg tds will usually be given.

- Diuretics: may be helpful if there is any evidence of fluid overload.

- Physiotherapy: to help with sputum expectoration, but will not be helpful if the patient has a very tight chest and is not coughing anything up.

If the patient does not improve with instigation of these treatments, then seek help sooner rather than later. Nasal intermittent positive-pressure ventilation and/or continuous positive airway pressure may be necessary, and endotracheal intubation and mechanical ventilation will be indicated in some patients. Decisions about such escalation of treatment are not straightforward. If confronted with a moribund patient in whom a decision has not already been made, then the default position must clearly be to proceed with treatment. However, no effort should be spared in discussing management with a respiratory physician if circumstances permit, preferably one who already knows the patient.

1.2.13 Stridor

Scenario

A 64-year-old woman who is a lifelong heavy smoker is brought to the Emergency Department with a history of progressive shortness of breath and 'noisy breathing'. She has been unwell for a couple of months, complains of generalised lethargy and weakness, and has lost weight. You are asked to see her urgently as the triage nurse thinks she has stridor.

Introduction

> **Priorities in the management of suspected stridor**
>
> - Check airway, breathing and circulation (ABC).
> - Get help early: you need someone with anaesthetic skills and possibly ear, nose and throat expertise.
> - Give 100% oxygen and obtain intravenous access.
> - Do *not* attempt to look at the patient's airway in any greater detail than carefully looking in the front of the mouth for any obvious blockage (eg dental plate); do *not* ask the patient to open his or her mouth as wide as possible; and do *not* put your fingers in 'hunting for something'.
> - Let patients determine their best position: often patients are sitting up, trying to manage their own airway. Getting them to lie flat may quickly change a borderline airway to a blocked one.
> - Consider the presumptive diagnosis (Table 4) and start treatment based on this.

History of the presenting problem

The patient may not be able to speak, in which case history may be available from someone else, but important features to consider include the following.

Speed of onset

Aspiration of a foreign body may present suddenly with a history

TABLE 4 CAUSES OF STRIDOR

Cause	Common example	Less common or rare example
Intrinsic narrowing of airway	Aspiration of a foreign body Anaphylaxis Epiglottitis (especially in children) Laryngeal tumour	Acute pharyngitis/laryngitis/ retropharyngeal abscess Laryngeal trauma Inhalation injury
Extrinsic compression of airway	Mediastinal tumour Retrosternal thyroid	Mediastinal lymphadenopathy

of coughing or choking; in acute anaphylaxis stridor is of sudden onset and can be quickly progressive; progressive hoarseness and shortness of breath with systemic deterioration (as in this case) are more suggestive of an underlying tumour; and patients with retrosternal thyroid enlargement may present with slow onset of dysphagia and hoarseness that pre-date the presentation of stridor.

Exacerbating or triggering factors

- Although not likely in this case with a history that seems to be of 2 months' duration, is there a history of a bee sting or other allergen exposure that may result in anaphylaxis?

- Is there a history of smoke inhalation, which may cause laryngeal oedema and bronchospasm within 48 hours of exposure?

- Is there a history of a prodromal viral/infective illness or sore throat that could suggest acute laryngitis or epiglottitis?

- Is there a history of intubation, bronchoscopy or laryngoscopy, all of which may result in laryngeal trauma, oedema or spasm?

- Is there a history of previous neck surgery or tracheostomy?

Other relevant history

Is there a history of known malignancy? This may be the first presentation of this patient with this malignancy, but it is important to find out if there is a history of thoracic or laryngeal malignancy, either of which may have progressed. Does the patient have a condition that could cause recurrent aspiration, eg motor neuron disease or progressive supranuclear palsy?

Examination

> 🔑 If the patient is *in extremis*, put out a cardiac arrest call immediately.

If the patient has stridor but is clinically stable and does not seem to be in danger of imminent catastrophe, then look for the following.

- Clubbing: would strongly suggest a malignant cause in this clinical context.

- Lymphadenopathy: enlarged cervical lymph nodes may be present in malignancy.

- Evidence of trauma: bruising or palpable subcutaneous crepitus in the neck.

- Signs of thyrotoxicosis, thyroid enlargement or the presence of a retrosternal thyroid.

- Distended and non-pulsatile neck veins: suggests superior vena cava obstruction.

- Rheumatoid arthritis: consider cricoarytenoid ankylosis.

Investigation

> ⚠️ If the patient has stridor and is in respiratory distress, then do not delay treatment and senior input while waiting for the results of investigations. Quick action to stabilise the airway and maintain adequate oxygenation is vital to prevent catastrophe.

If the patient is in a fit enough state to enable investigation, then the following are most likely to be helpful in revealing the diagnosis.

Routine haematological and biochemical screening tests should also be performed.

- CXR: may demonstrate evidence of underlying malignancy, mediastinal enlargement (lymphadenopathy/mediastinal tumour) or retrosternal thyroid. A lateral neck radiograph may also be informative.

- Nasoendoscopy: the investigation of choice in a patient with unexplained stridor. It should be performed by an experienced operator with appropriate anaesthetic cover in the event of deterioration. May demonstrate the presence of oedema, inflammation, foreign body, mucus plugging or tumour.

- Bronchoscopy: enables visualisation of the trachea and bronchi, which may enable diagnosis and therapeutic intervention.

- CT scan of the neck and thorax: may determine the level and cause of the obstruction, but not an investigation that can be performed without securing the airway if there is significant compromise.

- Flow–volume loops: useful when the cause of breathlessness is not obvious in order to establish whether there is upper airway obstruction.

Management

> 🔑 In patients with life-threatening stridor the priority is to gain control of the airway: this may necessitate intubation or tracheotomy (to bypass upper airway obstruction) before any further intervention.

Treat the following conditions on suspicion.

- Laryngeal oedema: give nebulised epinephrine (adrenaline) 5 mL of 1 in 1,000 solution (undiluted) and high-dose steroids (hydrocortisone 200 mg iv or dexamethasone 8–16 mg iv).
- Epiglottitis or laryngeal infection, or retropharyngeal abscess: give high-dose broad-spectrum intravenous antibiotics.

1.2.14 Pneumothorax

Scenario

You are called to the Emergency Department to review a 28-year-old man complaining of breathlessness and chest pain. On your arrival he is tachypnoeic, with pulse oximetry showing Sao_2 93% on an Fio_2 of 60%. His girlfriend tells you that about 4 hours ago he complained of right-sided chest pain followed by progressive breathlessness. He is on no regular medication and is a lifelong non-smoker. A CXR has just been done and confirms that he has a pneumothorax. How would you proceed?

Introduction

The first priority, as always, will be to make an assessment of the severity of illness, as described in Section 1.2.2, but the top priority in this case must clearly be to exclude tension pneumothorax.

Features of a tension pneumothorax

- The patient may be nearly dead.
- Cyanosis.

- Substantial respiratory effort (unless exhausted) but with little air movement.
- Chest looks 'blown up' on affected side.
- Tracheal deviation away from the affected side.
- Hyperresonance on percussion of the affected side.
- Absent breath sounds on the affected side.

Do not delay if you suspect tension pneumothorax: treat immediately

Insert a needle into the chest in the mid-axillary line on the affected side above the level of the nipple.

History of the presenting problem

In this case the diagnosis is already established, but in a less dramatic presentation the following features would suggest a diagnosis of acute spontaneous pneumothorax.

- Nature of onset of breathlessness: the patient is often able to pinpoint the exact time at which the breathlessness started, with sudden onset often in association with unilateral pleuritic chest pain. Many patients, particularly those with primary pneumothoraces (no evidence of coexisting lung disease), do not seek medical advice for several days.

- Chest pain: pleuritic pain results from damage to the pleural surfaces, and in conjunction with reduced ventilatory units (collapsed lung) can compromise gas exchange as a result of hypoventilation due to pain.

- Absence of fever or infective symptomatology: would argue against pneumonia being a cause of breathlessness and pleuritic chest pain.

Other relevant history

- Previous history of pneumothorax: the risk of recurrence of a primary

pneumothorax is about 50% within the first 4 years, with risk factors including smoking, height in male patients and age over 60 years. Risk factors for recurrence of secondary pneumothoraces include age, pulmonary fibrosis and emphysema.

- Smoking history: the risk of developing a pneumothorax is increased in smokers, with a lifetime risk of 12% in men that smoke compared with 0.1% in male non-smokers. The same trend is seen in women although to a lesser extent. The risk of recurrence is also higher in those who continue to smoke.

- Coexistent lung disease: the presence of coexisting lung disease, ie chronic obstructive pulmonary disease (COPD), will increase the risk of development of a pneumothorax (secondary pneumothorax) but will also have implications in relation to the ability of the patient to tolerate the complication. A relatively small pneumothorax may cause significant respiratory compromise in a patient with pre-existing lung disease.

Examination

The first priority is to exclude the presence of a tension pneumothorax. The signs may not be dramatic in a pneumothorax that is not under tension, but look specifically for reduced expansion, breath sounds, tactile vocal fremitus and vocal resonance on the affected side in association with a hyperresonant percussion note.

Also note any signs of associated lung pathology (eg COPD), which would not be expected in this young man, or any other predisposing condition, eg Marfan's syndrome.

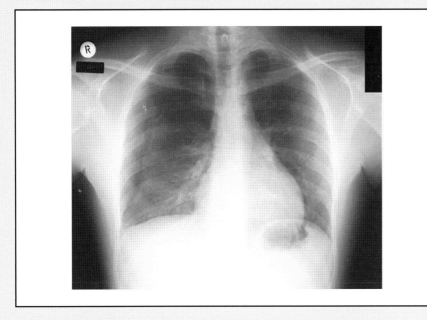

▲**Fig. 23** Large right-sided pneumothorax.

Investigation

This man with a primary (almost certainly) pneumothorax has already had the two key investigations: measurement of oxygen saturation and a CXR (Fig. 23). If the patient is very unwell or Sao_2 is <92%, then arterial blood gases should be checked to assess ventilation. In those with background lung disease, even a small pneumothorax may cause significant deterioration in oxygenation and hypercapnia.

When a pneumothorax is expected but not confirmed on the CXR, or it occurs in the presence of severe underlying emphysematous lung disease, then CT scanning is becoming an increasingly useful tool. It is vital that large bullae are not mistaken for an underlying pneumothorax.

What is a 'large' and what is a 'small' pneumothorax?

The British Thoracic Society (BTS) guidelines on pleural disease define this as follows.

- Small: a visible rim of air of <2 cm between the lung and the chest wall margin.
- Large: a visible rim of air >2 cm between the lung and the chest wall margin.

Management

The appropriate management will depend on the size of the pneumothorax, the degree of respiratory compromise and whether the patient has underlying respiratory problems.

- Small primary pneumothorax without significant breathlessness: observation alone is recommended. Patients with small primary pneumothoraces and minimal symptoms do not require admission to hospital, but it should be made clear to them that if they develop any symptoms of breathlessness or chest pain they should return to hospital immediately.

- Small secondary pneumothorax without significant breathlessness:

observation alone is appropriate in those with a pneumothorax <1 cm in depth, but hospitalisation is recommended in all cases.

Intervention is required for all patients with either primary or secondary pneumothoraces who are symptomatic, and in all patients with large pneumothoraces. All these patients require oxygen and adequate analgesia. Inhalation of a high concentration of oxygen increases the rate of resolution/air reabsorption four-fold every 24 hours. It is vitally important to maintain adequate analgesia to enable the patient to ventilate without pain and thus encourage re-expansion.

- Simple aspiration: this is recommended as first-line treatment for all primary pneumothoraces requiring intervention. In patients with secondary pneumothoraces it is only recommended as initial treatment in small cases with minimal symptoms, and if treatment is successful it is recommended that these patients be observed in hospital for 24 hours prior to discharge.

- Intercostal chest drain: should be inserted if simple aspiration fails (see Section 3.3), and is recommended in most patients with secondary pneumothoraces. There is no evidence that large tubes (28–32Fr) are any better than small tubes (12–14Fr), so use a small-bore tube initially, although this may have to be replaced with a larger tube if there is a persistent air leak.

Failure of a pneumothorax to re-expand after 48 hours requires specialist respiratory referral. High-pressure low-volume suction (–5 to –15 cmH$_2$O) may need to be considered. Surgical referral should be made at 5–7 days for those with a persistent air leak, and earlier in those with pre-existing lung disease who have a greater potential for complications.

Further comments

Patients discharged without intervention should be asked to reattend for a repeat CXR in 10–14 days. In all other patients resolution of the pneumothorax should be confirmed on a CXR prior to discharge, with further follow-up in 4–6 weeks.

The BTS Air Travel Working Party suggests that patients may travel safely by air 6 weeks after the resolution of a pneumothorax on CXR. There is still a significant risk of recurrence up to 1 year after resolution depending on whether the patient has an underlying lung disease, and because of this some patients may decide to avoid increasing the risk by not flying for a year.

Diving should be discouraged permanently after a pneumothorax unless a definitive surgical intervention has been performed.

1.2.15 Upper gastrointestinal haemorrhage

Scenario
A 70-year-old woman is brought to hospital having collapsed in her home. On arrival of the ambulance she was hypotensive (BP 82/44 mmHg), cold and sweaty. The ambulance crew report that there was evidence that she had vomited blood at home, and that she did so again whilst en route. You are asked to assess her urgently.

Introduction

> 🔑 This woman is clearly extremely unwell: your first priority must be to initiate resuscitation (see Section 1.2.2). Only when resuscitation is underway should your attention move towards trying to work out the cause of her haematemesis.

History of the presenting problem

This woman is most unlikely to be able to give much of a history at the moment, but in a patient who was less ill the following information should be sought.

- Has she vomited blood before and if so what was the cause?

- Has she had a peptic ulcer in the past?

- Is there a history of heartburn, dyspepsia, use of medications for indigestion or previous barium meal/endoscopy that might point to peptic ulcer disease?

- What medications is she on? Enquire about both prescribed and over-the-counter medications; take note of anticoagulants, NSAIDs and steroids in particular.

- Has she had liver disease in the past or is she at risk of this? After explaining why you need to know this information, ask in particular about alcohol intake: 'Are you a heavy drinker now or have you ever been in the past?' (See *Clinical Skills for PACES*.)

- Has there been recent weight loss, dysphagia or an early feeling of fullness when eating that might point to a malignancy?

> ⚠️ Are you sure the problem is haematemesis? In this case there does not seem to be any doubt, but patients often report that they have had 'dark vomit' and this might not be due to haematemesis. Keep an open mind to alternative diagnoses until haematemesis is proven.

Examination

The overall condition of the patient and the circulation should be assessed as described in Section 1.2.2, but with regard to someone with upper gastrointestinal bleeding note the following in addition.

- Signs of chronic liver disease or portal hypertension (Table 5 and Fig. 24).

TABLE 5 PHYSICAL SIGNS IN PATIENTS WITH LIVER DISEASE		
Signs of chronic liver disease	**Signs of portal hypertension**	**Signs of hepatic encephalopathy**
Spider naevi	Splenomegaly	Myoclonic jerks: the 'liver flap'
Palmar erythema	Ascites	Hepatic fetor
Leuconychia	Caput medusae	Impaired conscious level
Clubbing (rarely)		
Jaundice		
Bruising		
Scratch marks		
Gynaecomastia		
Loss of secondary sexual hair		
Testicular atrophy		

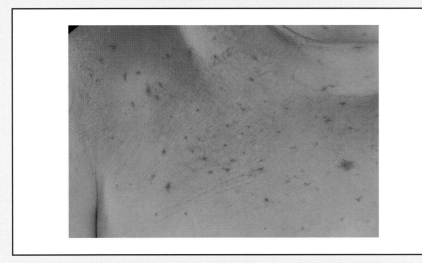

▲**Fig. 24** Spider naevi in a patient with alcohol-induced cirrhosis.

- Signs suggesting chronic iron deficiency anaemia: pale conjunctivae, smooth tongue, angular stomatitis and koilonychia.

- Signs of malignancy: look for Virchow's node and/or an epigastric mass.

- Digital rectal examination: look for melaena.

- Signs of aspiration.

Do not forget the rarities: finding subcutaneous emphysema in a patient with a history of severe vomiting is suggestive of Boerhaave's syndrome (oesophageal rupture) and requires prompt consideration of surgical therapy; telangiectasiae may indicate Osler–Weber–Rendu syndrome.

Investigation

Blood tests

This woman has clearly had a large bleed: arrange emergency cross-match of 4 units of her blood; group and save them in a case without haemodynamic disturbance. FBC, clotting screen, electrolytes, and renal and liver function tests are also required. Remember that a relatively normal haemoglobin does not exclude significant haemorrhage because there may have been insufficient time for haemodilution to have taken place; an iron-deficient picture suggests acute-on-chronic blood loss.

Other tests

CXR (portable; perform upright if the patient is very ill) if there is suspicion of aspiration. An abdominal film is extremely unlikely to provide diagnostic help in cases of gastrointestinal bleeding if there is no evidence of concomitant peritonism or intestinal obstruction: do not ask for one unless these are plausible diagnoses. An ECG is also necessary to look for coronary ischaemia/infarction precipitated by hypotension.

Tests to determine the cause of bleeding

The definitive investigation for haematemesis, which can also be therapeutic, is upper gastrointestinal endoscopy (Fig. 25). This should be performed after resuscitation of any patient who has had a significant haematemesis or, in skilled hands, while resuscitation is ongoing in the patient who is continuing to bleed.

> ⚠ It is not safe to endoscope a patient who is shocked and hypotensive.

> ⚠ Remember that upper gastrointestinal bleeding in the setting of alcohol abuse is often caused by a pathology other than oesophageal or gastric varices.

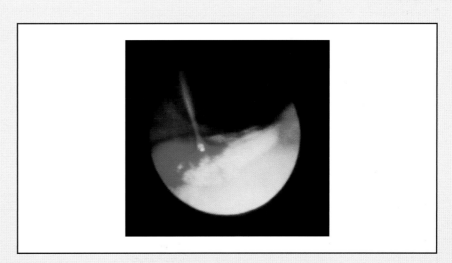

▲**Fig. 25** Endoscopy showing a peptic ulcer with a spurting artery: an obvious case for intervention.

Management

> Gastrointestinal bleeding is a team game: if haemorrhage is profuse, continuing or recurrent, get a surgical opinion sooner rather than later.

The immediate priority is to resuscitate (see Section 1.2.2), but note the following in particular.

- Establish venous access: insert large cannulae into both antecubital fossae. If access is difficult, insert a line into the femoral vein (which lies medial to the artery, as remembered by the acronym 'NAVY': nerve, artery, vein and Y-fronts). If you cannot do this, get someone who can.

> Never attempt central venous cannulation of a neck vein in a collapsed hypovolaemic patient because the veins are constricted, rendering the procedure difficult. Insertion of a central line has never made anyone better, but it has killed.

- Give intravenous fluids: 1 L of 0.9% saline as fast as possible while waiting for blood to arrive; then repeat the examination of pulse rate, BP and JVP. If hypotension persists and the JVP remains low, give more fluid rapidly (blood if available, or 0.9% saline) until the JVP is raised to the upper limit of normal and postural hypotension is abolished.

- Insert urinary catheter ('the poor man's central venous pressure'): a good urine output is a much better marker of the restoration of organ perfusion than measurement of central venous pressure.

- Proton pump inhibitors: omeprazole 80 mg iv bolus followed by infusion of 8 mg/hour for 72 hours has been shown to reduce the early rebleed rate in peptic ulcer with haemorrhage.

Further comment

Risk scoring in upper gastrointestinal haemorrhage

Haematemesis is a more serious symptom than melaena: mortality rises from 5% in patients suffering melaena with clear nasogastric aspirate to 12% in those with melaena and fresh blood in the nasogastric aspirate; patients passing red blood per rectum with fresh blood in the nasogastric aspirate are reported to have a mortality rate of 29%; older patients have a higher mortality; and the mortality of all patients who rebleed in hospital is 40%.

A combination of clinical features and endoscopic findings has provided a numerical scoring system of risk in upper gastrointestinal haemorrhage (Table 6), the maximum additive score prior to diagnosis by endoscopy being 7.

Varices

Bleeding oesophageal varices can cause a torrential loss of blood. Get specialist help immediately if this is likely to be the diagnosis. Urgent endoscopy is mandatory: banding or sclerotherapy can be attempted during the procedure. Consider giving terlipressin to try to reduce portal BP (2 mg iv, followed by 1 or 2 mg every 4–6 hours until bleeding is controlled, for up to 72 hours). Have a Sengstaken–Blakemore tube available, but this should only be used by those with experience of the technique. Patients with massive bleeding should be considered for intubation to reduce the increased risk of aspiration. Surgical treatment

TABLE 6 RISK SCORING SYSTEM FOR ACUTE UPPER GASTROINTESTINAL BLEEDING

Score	0	1	2	3
Age	<60 years	60–79 years	>80 years	
Shock	No shock	Pulse >100 bpm with systolic BP >100 mmHg	Systolic BP <100 mmHg	
Comorbidity	None		Cardiac failure, ischaemic heart disease and other major comorbidities	Renal failure, liver failure and widespread malignancy
Diagnosis	Mallory–Weiss tear or no lesion seen	All other diagnoses	Malignancy of upper gastrointestinal tract	
Major stigmata of recent haemorrhage at endoscopy	None or dark spot only		Blood in upper gastrointestinal tract, adherent clot visible or spurting vessel	

Mortality rate by additive score is as follows: score 0, 0.2%; score 1, 2.4%; score 2, 5.6%; score 3, 11%; score 4, 25%; score 5, 40%; score 6 or 7, 50%.

for acute variceal bleeding is rarely done because of high mortality, but the TIPS (transjugular intrahepatic portosystemic shunt) procedure can be considered in some cases.

1.2.16 Bloody diarrhoea

Scenario

A 37-year-old woman is sent to the Medical Assessment Unit by her GP with a 48-hour history of frequent watery diarrhoea; blood has been mixed with the motions for the past 24 hours, during which time she has had her bowels open ten times. You are asked to review her.

History of the presenting problem

Intensity and nature of the diarrhoea

- Has the patient got diarrhoea at all? The history seems clear-cut in this case, but patients use the term 'diarrhoea' to describe different things. How many times has she opened her bowels today? Be aware that a sudden fall in

stool frequency can indicate acute colonic dilatation and subsequent perforation.

- What is the nature of the diarrhoea? Frequent passage of small amounts of stool suggests proctitis or a rectal lesion; large volumes indicate small-bowel pathology. Bloody diarrhoea is very suggestive of colonic pathology, whereas copious foul-smelling bulky stools that are difficult to flush away are characteristic of malabsorption.

- Is there diarrhoea at night? This is useful in distinguishing irritable bowel syndrome from organic pathology.

Physiology of the bowel

The daily dietary intake of food and liquid combined with gastric and intestinal secretions results in a volume load of about 7 L entering the small intestine. By the time intestinal contents have reached the terminal ileum, only about 1.5 L remains, so small-bowel pathology often causes large-volume diarrhoea.

Precipitating factors

Consider infectious causes: has the patient eaten any food that she thinks may have been contaminated or infected? Has anyone else that she knows had a similar problem? Has she been abroad recently? Clues to specific intestinal infections in the patient presenting with diarrhoea are shown in Table 7. Also ask about medication: has she taken antibiotics recently, which predispose to *Clostridium difficile*? Has she taken NSAIDs? These are a potent cause of colonic irritation and bloody diarrhoea.

Other relevant history

Has there been a previous history of bowel problems (could this be a flare of known inflammatory bowel disease?), bowel surgery or abdominal irradiation ('radiation colitis' can present with bloody diarrhoea). Is there any other relevant pathology? The sudden onset of pain and bloody diarrhoea in an elderly arteriopath should alert you to the possibility of ischaemic colitis.

The possibility of sexually transmitted infections and HIV-related infection must be considered

TABLE 7 CLUES TO PARTICULAR INTESTINAL INFECTIONS		
Site of infection	Infectious agent	Predisposing cause
Small-bowel infection	Cholera	Foreign travel
	Enterotoxigenic *Escherichia coli*	Infected meat
	Rotavirus, Norwalk virus, small round virus	Common and associated with vomiting
	Toxin-producing *Staphylococcus aureus*	Symptoms a few hours after ingestion of contaminated material; associated with vomiting
	Toxin-producing *Bacillus cereus*	Classically associated with contaminated rice and accompanied by vomiting
	Campylobacter jejuni	Commonest infectious cause in the UK today; beware of undercooked chicken
Colonic infection	*Shigella* and *Salmonella*	Classical cause of dysentery and associated with bloody diarrhoea
	Amoebiasis	Can be contracted in UK, so an important consideration on acute medical 'intake'
	Clostridium difficile	Associated with antibiotic therapy; toxin producing
	Enterohaemorrhagic *E. coli*	Produces a shiga-like toxin; can cause haemolytic–uraemic syndrome

if the diagnosis does not become apparent, in which case it will be necessary to take a sexual history. As always, this must be done with tact: explain why you need the information before asking for it and proceed carefully, as indicated in *Clinical Skills for PACES*.

Examination

The overall condition of the patient and the circulation should be assessed as described in Section 1.2.2, but in someone with bloody diarrhoea take particular note of the following.

- General features: fever, nutritional status and anaemia.

- Abdomen: distension, peritonism, masses and character of bowel sounds.

- Digital rectal examination: inspect the perineum first, looking for skin changes or fistulae suggestive of Crohn's disease; palpate for a rectal mass; and examine any faeces for melaena or frank blood.

Investigation

Cultures

Faeces should be sent for microbiological investigation (microscopy, culture and specific testing for *Clostridium difficile* toxin); the sample can be obtained during sigmoidoscopy if the patient has not been able to provide one before this is performed. Also test blood cultures.

Radiology

An erect CXR should include the hemidiaphragms to look for evidence of perforation (Fig. 26). A supine abdominal film should be taken to exclude toxic dilatation and to look for mucosal islands and a dilated small bowel, which are other adverse prognostic radiological signs of inflammatory bowel disease (Fig. 27).

Sigmoidoscopy

Sigmoidoscopy (Fig. 28) should be performed after the abdominal radiograph because introduction of air during the procedure can produce a picture alarmingly similar to toxic dilatation. Normal rectal mucosa usually excludes active ulcerative colitis. Inflamed rectal mucosa can be a feature of any cause of severe diarrhoea. The mucosal appearance of *Clostridium difficile* infection is also variable, although the adherent yellow-white plaques, or 'pseudomembrane', is characteristic. A rectal biopsy should be taken below the peritoneal reflection, ie within 10 cm of the anal margin.

Blood tests

- FBC may show acute anaemia, but it is more likely to indicate chronic pathology, eg poorly controlled inflammatory bowel disease. The blood film and haematological indices are important: microcytic hypochromic changes are likely to indicate blood loss, whereas macrocytosis points to malabsorption or alcohol abuse. A slight elevation in white cell count is of little help in differential diagnosis, but if the count is greater than 15×10^9/L consider sepsis.

- Electrolytes and renal/liver/bone profiles: severe diarrhoea can cause profound hypokalaemia.

- Serum albumin <30 g/L is a bad feature in inflammatory bowel disease because albumin loss is proportional to the extent of bowel involvement.

- Inflammatory markers: check C-reactive protein (CRP).

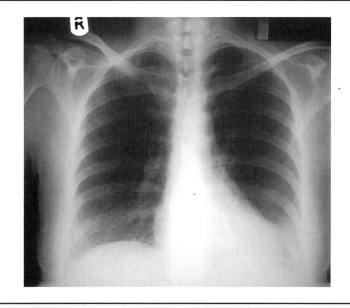

▲**Fig. 26** CXR showing air under both hemidiaphragms. No apologies for the subtle changes: they are often as subtle in real life!

Findings of concern in acute ulcerative colitis

- Bowels open 9–12 times in the first 24 hours.
- Pulse >100 bpm.

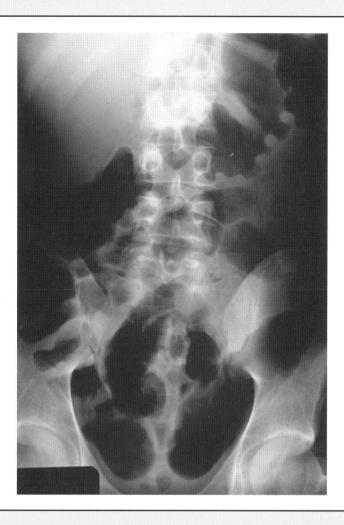

- Fever >38°C.
- Albumin <30 g/L.
- CRP >45 mg/L.
- Mucosal islands, toxic megacolon and dilated small bowel on abdominal radiograph.

▲**Fig. 27** Abdominal radiograph in acute ulcerative colitis. The colon is dilated (not quite to 10 cm, but worrying nonetheless). Thumb-printing of colonic mucosa is seen in the left upper abdomen and there are dilated loops of small bowel.

Management

Resuscitation, if required, will as always be the immediate priority (see Section 1.2.2). Specific management will depend on the cause of the problem, but note the following.

- Infective colitis: must be considered in all cases of acute colitis. If the patient is very ill and you cannot exclude infection, then it is safer to treat empirically with a combination of ciprofloxacin and metronidazole. This will cover most potential pathogens, including amoebae and *Clostridium difficile*.

- Pseudomembranous colitis: associated with antibiotic usage, particularly third-generation cephalosporins. Treat with metronidazole (iv or po) or vancomycin (po) after sigmoidoscopy (and rectal biopsy) has been performed and stool has been sent for *Clostridium difficile* toxin.

- Inflammatory bowel disease: a moderate or severe exacerbation should be treated with systemic steroids (eg methylprednisolone 80–120 mg iv daily given in two divided doses). Less severe exacerbations (perhaps limited to the rectum) may be appropriately managed with rectal steroid preparations, with or without a smaller dose of oral or intravenous steroid. 5-Aminosalicylic acid products may also have a role in management of the acute attack.

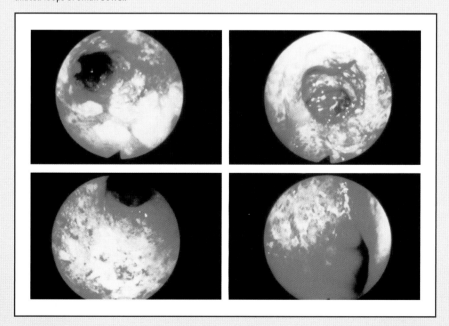

▲**Fig. 28** Sigmoidoscopic appearances of ulcerative colitis, showing inflamed mucosa, ulceration and contact bleeding.

> ⚠️ In patients with known inflammatory bowel disease, early involvement of the colorectal surgical team is mandatory: do not wait until there is radiographic evidence of toxic megacolon or perforation.

1.2.17 Abdominal pain

Scenario

A 42-year-old woman is referred to the Emergency Department with epigastric and back pain that has progressively worsened over the preceding 48 hours. She has been unable to eat for the last 24 hours because of nausea and vomiting, and she is in significant discomfort. The on-call surgeon has seen her and said that 'the problem is not surgical', so she has been referred to the medical team and you are asked to assess her.

Introduction

> 🔑 Patients do not know whether their abdominal pain is 'surgical' or 'medical': as a physician you must be wary of the acute abdomen that has been incorrectly referred, those conditions that may require joint management (eg biliary tract diseases) and the rare medical mimics of a 'surgical abdomen' (basal pneumonia, atypical presentation of myocardial infarction, diabetic ketoacidosis and porphyria).

History of the presenting problem

Onset and time course of pain

Most cases of abdominal pain start gradually, but perforation of a viscus can occasionally cause sudden pain.

The pain of duodenal ulceration is typically severe in the early hours of the morning, and there may be a definite periodicity to the pain, ie nightly bouts of pain for a few weeks followed by a symptom-free period. Severe acute pain persisting for several hours often implies a catastrophic event such as perforation, strangulation or intestinal obstruction.

Biliary pain often becomes more intense with time, but can be relieved suddenly with the passage of a stone.

Precipitating or relieving factors

Pain from the parietal peritoneum is exacerbated by even slight movement, which explains why patients with peritonitis lie perfectly still. In contrast, visceral pain often causes the patient to writhe around in an attempt to find a more comfortable position when a spasm of pain attacks.

Relief of pain by food is a strong pointer to peptic ulceration. Exacerbation by food implies an obstructive component, gastritis or oesophagitis. Gastric or duodenal inflammation is associated with alcohol, aspirin and other NSAIDs. Diffuse abdominal pain appearing 2 minutes to 1 hour after a meal raises the possibility of intestinal angina. Oesophageal pain is typically brought on by bending or stooping. Pain aggravated by tension or anxiety is a feature of irritable bowel syndrome.

Nature and distribution of pain

Constant, generalised and severe pain that is exacerbated by any movement is highly suggestive of peritonitis. Colicky pain is likely to be visceral in origin. The site where visceral pain is experienced depends on the intestinal segment involved: oesophageal pain is often in the epigastrium or low central chest; duodenal pain is felt in the epigastrium or just to the right of it; small bowel pain is poorly localised and is generally felt diffusely in the periumbilical region; and colonic pain usually occurs in roughly the area of the diseased colonic segment. Pain that is maximal in the right upper quadrant points to biliary tract disease, and pain sited in the flank with radiation to the anterior abdomen and inguinal region is suggestive of renal colic. Pancreatic pain is sited in the epigastrium, but there is often a lot of associated discomfort in the lumbar region of the back; pancreatitis is also a potential cause of generalised abdominal pain, which can mimic the peritonism of a ruptured viscus.

> ⚠️ Patients must not be denied analgesia, but once this has been given the nature and distribution of pain may change dramatically.

Referral of pain

Pain may be referred from visceral organs or the parietal peritoneum to areas innervated by the same dermatome: oesophageal pain may radiate to the neck and arms; gallbladder pain radiates to the right infrascapular region, where there may be hyperaesthesia over the referred area; and pain from a duodenal ulcer that radiates through to the back usually indicates penetration of the ulcer into the pancreas.

> 🔑 Be wary of thoracic pathology masquerading as an acute abdomen: pleurisy of the lower pleural surfaces can result in referred pain in the upper abdomen.

Associated symptoms

A full functional enquiry related to the abdomen is clearly required. This woman has been vomiting: how often, what, how much and does it relieve the pain? How are her bowels? Have these been normal, when was the last bowel motion and was it normal? Has she had any urinary symptoms such as frequency, dysuria, haematuria and pneumaturia? When was her last period and was it normal? Has she been feverish? And as a marker of longer-standing illness, has she lost any weight recently?

Other relevant history

- Drugs: codeine- or morphine-based drugs predispose to constipation with or without subacute obstruction. NSAIDs predispose to peptic ulceration. Oral contraceptives may increase the risk of gallstone formation.

- Alcohol: acute abdominal pain in alcoholics may result from gastritis, peptic ulceration, acute pancreatitis, tense ascites or spontaneous bacterial peritonitis.

- Past medical history: always ask if there is any history of similar presentations, and if so what diagnosis has been established (if any). Previous abdominal operations raise the possibility of adhesions that can cause intestinal obstruction. Comorbid illnesses may also be relevant in both diagnosis (eg the patient with widespread arterial disease is more likely to have an ischaemic gut) and in assessing the fitness of the patient for surgery (should it be a management option).

Examination

The overall condition of the patient and the circulation should be assessed as described in Section 1.2.2, but in someone with acute abdominal pain note the following in particular.

- Inspection: how does the patient appear? Dead, nearly dead, in pain, lying still or writhing around? Is she holding her abdomen rigidly? Is the abdomen distended or are there any obvious masses? Is there any bruising of the body wall that may occur with pancreatitis, ie umbilical (Cullen's sign) or in the flanks (Grey Turner's sign)?

- Palpation: is there peritonism? Are there localised abdominal findings, eg local tenderness with or without a mass, an enlarged organ, or perhaps a pyonephrosis or an empyema of the gallbladder? Always examine the hernial orifices, remembering to look carefully in unusual sites, eg periumbilical.

- Auscultation: are the bowel sounds normal or do they sound obstructed? Is there complete silence suggesting peritonitis?

- Digital rectal examination: this may reveal hard stool in the elderly, compacted and obstructed patient; or the rectum may be empty as in small bowel obstruction. Tenderness in the right iliac fossa on rectal examination is common in patients with appendicitis.

Look specifically for cachexia and/or enlarged supraclavicular lymph nodes, suggesting malignancy, and also for evidence of chronic liver disease (see Section 1.2.15).

Investigation

> The patient with obvious peritonism requires immediate resuscitation, analgesia, urgent surgical review and a laparotomy.

Blood tests

- FBC: anaemia may indicate chronic gastrointestinal blood loss; elevated white cell count may be due to pancreatitis.

- Electrolytes and renal/liver/bone profiles: look for hypokalaemia due to vomiting, renal impairment, raised urea in upper gastrointestinal blood loss and/or dehydration; an abnormal liver profile may indicate a biliary cause for the presentation; and elevated serum calcium may in rare cases explain the patient's abdominal pain.

- Amylase: must be checked without fail. A raised serum amylase can be seen in acute cholecystitis and in peptic ulceration, but if serum amylase is five times greater than normal then pancreatitis is likely.

- Note C-reactive protein, which will be non-specific if raised but reassuring if normal.

- Blood glucose: acute diabetic ketoacidosis can present with abdominal pain.

Imaging

- Erect CXR: better at diagnosing perforation than an abdominal film and may also show unexpected lower lobe pathology (pneumonia or collapse due to splinting of the diaphragm).

- Supine abdominal radiograph: may diagnose intestinal obstruction or help to localise pathology, eg the dilated contiguous loop of bowel in cholecystitis, the pattern of bowel dilatation seen with sigmoid volvulus or the classical appearances of toxic megacolon. Look for biliary or renal stones. Is there pancreatic calcification suggestive of previous pancreatitis?

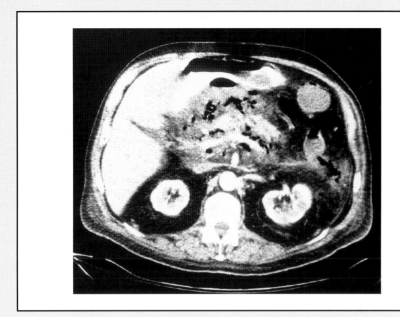

▲**Fig. 29** CT scan showing necrotising pancreatitis with gas formation. The patient had presented with abdominal pain indistinguishable from that due to peritonitis.

- Abdominal ultrasonography: helpful if you suspect biliary disease.

- Abdominal CT scan: you should not delay surgical intervention in the patient with obvious peritonitis to perform this, but it is a very useful and increasingly used investigation (Fig. 29).

Other investigations

If there is clinical suspicion of infection, examine blood cultures, urine cultures and stool cultures. If the patient is very ill, measure arterial blood gases to check for metabolic acidosis and that oxygenation and ventilation are adequate; also check the lactate level.

Management

> The on-call surgeon has said that this patient does not have a 'surgical abdomen', but if you disagree talk with him or her and get senior review.

Resuscitation, if required, will as always be the immediate priority (see Section 1.2.2). Specific management will depend on the cause of the problem, but note the following.

- Nil by mouth with or without a nasogastric tube: a nasogastric tube should be placed to clear the stomach contents if the patient continues to vomit or there is evidence of obstruction. The patient should remain nil by mouth until a diagnosis and management plan have been formulated.

- Urinary catheter: close monitoring of urine output is essential in any patient who is critically unwell.

- Antibiotics: if there is evidence of sepsis then broad-spectrum antibiotics should be given promptly after cultures have been taken, guided by microbiological advice and local policy.

Further comments

Very rare causes of an acute abdomen include the following.

- Acute intermittent porphyria: an inborn error of the synthesis of haem, resulting in overproduction of the intermediate compounds called porphyrins. Commonly presents around 30 years of age with abdominal pain, vomiting and constipation.

- Diabetic ketoacidosis.

- Sickle cell crisis: vaso-occlusive problems may occur in the small vessels of any organs including the spleen, liver, kidneys and bowel.

- Familial Mediterranean fever: characterised by recurrent attacks of fever, arthritis and abdominal or chest pain.

1.2.18 Hepatic encephalopathy/alcohol withdrawal

Scenario

A 65-year-old woman is brought to the Emergency Department having been found confused and shaking in her flat. She is known to be an alcoholic and attends the Emergency Department regularly. Her warden told the ambulance crew that she had been vomiting recently.

Introduction

Your main concern in an alcoholic patient who presents with confusion and tremor is to exclude any serious or life-threatening condition. Do not assume that the patient is just drunk: this is a dangerous thing to do, both for you and for the patient. Consider the differential diagnosis (Table 8) as you gather the history.

TABLE 8 DIFFERENTIAL DIAGNOSIS OF CONFUSION IN AN ALCOHOLIC

Cause	Condition
Specifically alcohol related	Alcohol intoxication Acute alcohol withdrawal Delirium tremens Wernicke's encephalopathy
Acute-on-chronic liver failure	Hypoglycaemia Hepatic encephalopathy
Other cerebral	Subdural haematoma Post ictal
Other	Any severe illness, particularly sepsis Hypothermia

History of the presenting problem

Dealing with a 'confused' patient

- Make sure the problem is confusion and not dysarthria or dysphasia.
- Establish baseline score on Glasgow Coma Scale (Fig. 40).
- Establish baseline score on Abbreviated Mental Test.

! If you cannot get a history from the patient, you must try to get one from somebody else.

Abbreviated Mental Test Score

Each question scores 1 mark and the test is marked out of 10. No half marks are allowed. A score of 6 or below is likely to indicate impaired cognition.

1. Age?
2. Time (to nearest hour)?
3. Address for recall at end of test (eg 42 West Street).
4. What year is it?
5. Name of institution?
6. Recognition of two persons' identities (can the patient identify your job and that of a nurse?).
7. Date of birth (day and month)?
8. In what year did World War I begin?
9. Name of the present monarch?
10. Count backwards from 20 to 1.

This woman will not be able to give a reliable history, but ask questions of anyone who knows anything about her circumstances and explore factors that may precipitate acute deterioration in someone with known alcoholic liver disease (if there are none, call the warden to try to get further details).

- Binge drinking or acute alcohol withdrawal: how much alcohol does she usually drink? Has she stopped over the past few days or has she been on a 'bender': an extended drinking session that has become so excessive she is no longer able to function?

- Gastrointestinal disturbance: a gastrointestinal bleed may cause acute decompensation, as may constipation.

- Trauma/head injury: alcoholics frequently fall over.

- Infection: any infection may cause deterioration. Ask particularly about respiratory and urinary symptoms.

- Drug history: a wide range of drugs can cause liver problems, but note especially those that commonly cause decompensation of chronic liver disease, eg analgesics, benzodiazepines, opioids and diuretics.

Examination

Begin with an overall assessment as described in Section 1.2.2 before proceeding to note the following.

General features

- Smell: does she smell of alcohol or is there hepatic fetor?

- Evidence of hepatic encephalopathy: liver flap; grade severity (Table 9).

- Signs of chronic liver disease (see Section 1.2.15 and Fig. 30).

- Nutritional status.

Abdominal

Examine for tenderness, hepatomegaly (unlikely in chronic liver disease), splenomegaly and ascites. Rectal examination for melaena is essential.

Abdominal tenderness can be the first sign of spontaneous bacterial peritonitis in a patient with chronic liver disease.

TABLE 9 GRADES OF HEPATIC ENCEPHALOPATHY

Grade	Status
Grade 1	Mildly drowsy but coherent; mood change, impaired concentration and psychomotor function
Grade 2	Drowsy and confused, but able to answer questions
Grade 3	Very drowsy but rousable; alternatively incoherent and agitated
Grade 4a	Responsive only to painful stimuli
Grade 4b	Unresponsive

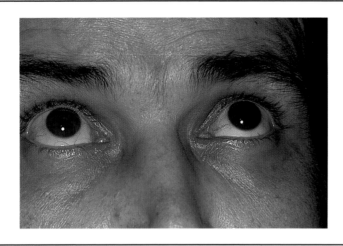

▲**Fig. 30** Always look carefully for jaundice. (Reproduced with permission from Axford J. *Medicine*. Oxford: Blackwell Science, 1996.)

Neurological

Aside from features of hepatic encephalopathy, look specifically for evidence of the following.

- Head injury/subdural haemorrhage: the risk of a subdural or extradural haematoma is high if the pupils are unequal or there are localising signs.

- Wernicke's encephalopathy.

- Korsakoff's syndrome: gross defect of memory for recent events, with gaps in memory filled by confabulation.

> **Wernicke's encephalopathy**
> - Ophthalmoplegia: horizontal and/or vertical nystagmus; weakness/failure of eye abduction; weakness/failure of conjugate gaze.
> - Ataxia.
> - Confusion.

Investigation

> Check fingerprick blood glucose to exclude hypoglycaemia.

Routine blood tests

Perform FBC, coagulation screen, electrolytes and renal/liver/bone profiles and measure glucose and an inflammatory marker (C-reactive protein). A wide range of abnormalities may be found.

Tests to look for infection

- Blood and urine cultures.

- CXR for signs of consolidation (check also for fractured ribs).

- If ascites is present, then tap to look for evidence of spontaneous bacterial peritonitis, which is diagnosed if this reveals a neutrophil count above 500×10^6/L.

Other investigations

Depending on the clinical context it may be appropriate to check serum amylase, perform arterial blood gases or organise a CT scan of the brain.

Management

> If there is a history of chronic alcohol intake or malnourishment, give thiamine before glucose to avoid precipitating

> Wernicke's encephalopathy. This is usually done by giving two pairs of ampoules of high-potency thiamine (Pabrinex) intravenously.

Specific management will clearly depend on the diagnosis (Table 8). However, if the working diagnosis is acute-on-chronic liver failure related to alcohol, then note the following.

Hypovolaemia and electrolyte disturbance

- Hypoglycaemia: give intravenous glucose to maintain fingerprick blood glucose >3.5 mmol/L (the patient may also require continuous infusion of 10% dextrose), but only after giving thiamine.

- Hypovolaemia: give colloid rather than the usual 0.9% saline.

- Hyponatraemia: this is common and is due to water excess not sodium deficiency; hence treat with water restriction and not with 0.9% saline.

- Hypokalaemia: give intravenous potassium.

- Hypophosphataemia: start intravenous or oral replacement therapy.

Feeding and gastric protection

- Nasogastric tube: adequate nutrition is important and drugs can be given reliably by this route.

- Ranitidine 50 mg iv three times daily to reduce the risk of stress ulceration.

Reduction of intestinal nitrogenous load

- Start lactulose 20–30 mL or lactitol 10 g three times daily, reducing the dose when diarrhoea starts.

- Give a phosphate enema.

- Consider giving neomycin or metronidazole if the patient is poorly responsive or comatose.

Coagulopathy

- Give vitamin K orally or intravenously (preferable).

- Consider giving fresh frozen plasma or platelets if the patient is actively bleeding.

Underlying infection

Start broad-spectrum antibiotics (eg ceftriaxone or cefotaxime 2 g iv twice daily) if infection is suspected. Remember that bacterial peritonitis occurs in around 25% of patients with cirrhotic ascites.

Vitamin supplementation

Vitamins B and C are usually deficient in chronic alcoholics. If consciousness is impaired, give intravenous thiamine (Pabrinex) two to three pairs of ampoules every 8 hours (this can cause anaphylaxis). If the patient can take oral medications, start oral thiamine (50 mg od), vitamin B compound tablets strong (one to two tablets tds) and vitamin C (100 mg od).

Anticipate and treat complications

> The development of complications indicates a very poor prognosis and it may be inappropriate to escalate treatment. This is an issue that requires careful consideration and discussion with senior colleagues. If in doubt, contact the regional liver centre for advice.

Renal failure is a common complication of liver failure. It is most frequently due to acute tubular necrosis, although the prognosis for hepatorenal syndrome is particularly

poor. Cerebral oedema is another feared complication: consider giving mannitol 200 mg/kg iv slowly; intracranial pressure monitoring can be useful but is not available in all centres.

Acute alcohol withdrawal and delirium tremens

> **Acute alcohol withdrawal**
>
> This is common; it typically causes tremor and confusion after 8–24 hours and settles after 48 hours.
>
> **Delirium tremens**
>
> This is rare, but can be fatal if untreated. Symptoms include tremor, confusion, visual hallucinations, fever and sweating; usually occurs 3–4 days after stopping drinking.

Aside from the standard supportive measures, give vitamins (as above), treat hypoglycaemia and prescribe sedation.

- If the patient can tolerate oral therapy, give chlordiazepoxide 30 mg four times on day 1, then treat with a reducing dose.

- If the patient is severely agitated and unable to take oral medications, give intravenous clomethiazole (chlormethiazole) 0.8% solution at an initial rate of 20–60 mg/min until shallow sleep (from which the patient can be easily roused) is induced. Then reduce the rate to the lowest possible to maintain shallow sleep and normal spontaneous respiration.

> ⚠ Clomethiazole can cause respiratory depression: patients must be closely monitored and full resuscitation facilities must be available.

1.2.19 Renal failure, fluid overload and hyperkalaemia

> ### Scenario
>
> A 67-year-old man had elective bilateral hip replacement 5 days ago. Over the last 24 hours he has become increasingly breathless and the observation charts show that no urine output has been recorded, which the nurse in charge of the ward confirms to be true. The orthopaedic doctor on duty asks the on-call medical team to review this patient urgently.

Introduction

The most likely explanation for this scenario is the development of postoperative acute or acute-on-chronic renal failure, and the most pressing concerns are that the patient might have hyperkalaemia and/or pulmonary oedema.

 Hyperkalaemia can kill suddenly and without warning.

Recognition of significant hyperkalaemia

A 12-lead ECG should be done in all acutely unwell patients: in this case this might reveal changes diagnostic of myocardial infarction or consistent with pulmonary embolism (PE), but the most important matter is to look for evidence of hyperkalaemia. The following ECG changes occur sequentially as the patient's serum potassium rises:

- tall 'peaked' T waves;

- flattened P waves, prolonged PR interval and wide QRS complexes;

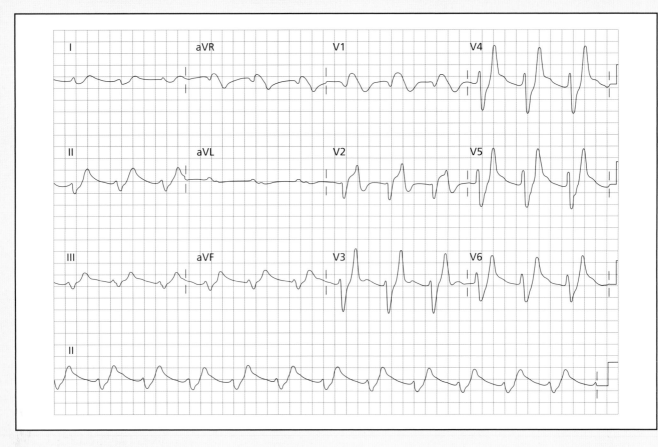

▲**Fig. 31** ECG changes in severe hyperkalaemia.

- absent P waves and very wide QRS complexes slurring into T waves (Fig. 31);

- cardiac arrest (ventricular fibrillation, ventricular tachycardia and asystole).

Urgent treatment is required if there is any change more severe than T-wave peaking; take a specimen for measurement of serum potassium, but do not wait for the result. It is not a triumph to be told that serum potassium was 9.1 mmol/L just after the patient has arrested.

Treatment of significant hyperkalaemia

If the patient's ECG looks like that shown in Fig. 31, give calcium immediately, followed by dextrose/insulin or salbutamol.

- Calcium gluconate 10% solution, 10 mL iv over 1–2 minutes. This does not lower the serum potassium level but reduces myocardial excitability. Its effect is instant, with the ECG becoming less abnormal in front of your eyes.

- Dextrose (50 mL of 50% solution) plus 10 units short-acting insulin, eg Actrapid (soluble insulin), intravenously over 15–30 minutes. This shifts potassium into the intracellular compartment. It should not cause hypoglycaemia, but check fingerprick blood glucose if in any doubt. Serum potassium falls by 1–2 mmol/L over 30–60 minutes.

- Salbutamol (nebulised) 10 mg: this activates the intracellular adenylate cyclase system and induces a shift of potassium into the intracellular compartment. Serum potassium falls by 1–2 mmol/L over 30–60 minutes.

Calcium, dextrose/insulin and salbutamol are holding measures only, reducing the serum potassium concentration for 4–6 hours. Most patients with severe hyperkalaemia require urgent haemodialysis, the exceptions being the few whose renal function improves rapidly, eg after relief of acute obstruction.

After giving emergency treatment for hyperkalaemia, do not forget to contact the intensive care unit (ICU) or local renal unit to arrange transfer for urgent haemofiltration or dialysis if the patient's urine output does not respond immediately and dramatically to fluid and/or bladder catheterisation.

Oral and rectal ion-exchange resins increase gut excretion of potassium and can be used to take the 'edge' off hyperkalaemia, but they take 24 hours to have any effect and are not an emergency treatment for hyperkalaemia.

History of the presenting problem

After considering and (if necessary) treating hyperkalaemia, consider causes of postoperative breathlessness as described in Section 1.2.5 and find out from the patient, medical records and/or observation charts if he has any history of renal/urinary problems (any symptoms of prostatism?) or pre-existing renal impairment (what was the preoperative serum creatinine?). Investigate precisely what happened to him during his operation and afterwards, noting vital signs (was he hypotensive at any time, which might explain acute tubular necrosis?), daily fluid input/output, administration of drugs and whether he now feels as though he wants to pass urine (acute retention).

Examination

Is this man ill, very ill or nearly dead? As always, begin with an overall assessment as described in Section 1.2.2, taking particular care to look for evidence of the following.

Pulmonary oedema

- Respiratory rate: tachypnoea would be expected and could indicate fluid overload, metabolic acidosis or pneumonia. Beware a low or normal respiratory rate in patients who you would expect to have a high rate, since they may have become exhausted and be about to die.

- Pulse rate and rhythm: the patient is likely to have tachycardia, but look particularly for fast atrial fibrillation, which is a common problem postoperatively.

- BP: may be elevated in pulmonary oedema.

- Jugular venous pulse: may be difficult to see, but expected to be high in fluid overload.

- Heart sounds: listen for gallop rhythm indicating that the left ventricle is under strain.

- Lungs: are there bilateral crackles suggesting fluid overload or (less likely) localised crackles or a pleural rub to suggest infection or PE?

Urinary retention

- Is the bladder palpable?

Investigation

As described in Section 1.2.5, with the following of particular note in addition to the ECG.

- Electrolytes and renal function tests: to confirm the presence of hyperkalaemia and/or renal failure.

- Serum troponin: has the stress of the operation precipitated a myocardial infarction?

- Consider sepsis: a common precipitant of postoperative renal failure; take relevant cultures.

- CXR: look at the heart size, and for pulmonary oedema or infection.

- Arterial blood gases: expect a partially compensated metabolic acidosis in a sick patient with renal failure. A normal $Pa\text{co}_2$ would probably be worrying in this case as it would indicate that the patient is getting tired and losing respiratory compensation, in which case acidosis can worsen very rapidly with dire consequences.

Management

If this man looks very ill or about to die, then call for help from ICU immediately. Otherwise, proceed as described in Section 1.2.2 and take particular care to do the following.

- Insert a urinary catheter: this will relieve outflow obstruction if present, which may result in a prompt diuresis and restoration of renal function.

- Stop nephrotoxins: NSAIDs (commonly used for postoperative analgesia), angiotensin-converting enzyme inhibitors and angiotensin receptor blockers all have adverse effects on renal blood flow in this context and should be (temporarily) stopped, as should aminoglycoside antibiotics.

Management of fluid overload in the patient with renal failure

- Sit the patient up.

- Give high-flow oxygen.

- Restrict fluid input to the minimum possible.

- Nitrate, eg isosorbide dinitrate 2–20 mg/hour iv, titrated to as high a dose as the BP will allow.

- Diuretic, eg furosemide 250 mg iv over 1 hour, may induce some increase in urine output.

- Dialysis/ultrafiltration: arrange urgently if the patient remains overloaded.

- Non-invasive ventilation/ continuous positive airway pressure: can be very effective in treating breathlessness due to pulmonary oedema.

⚠️ When inserting a central line for dialysis access in a patient with pulmonary oedema:

- do not lie the patient down since cardiac arrest is likely;
- do not use the subclavian vein because the patient will not tolerate a pneumothorax;
- use the femoral vein.

Indications for urgent dialysis

- Persistent hyperkalaemia.
- Refractory pulmonary oedema.
- Severe metabolic acidosis.
- Symptomatic uraemia, eg altered mental status, fits, asterixis and pericarditis.

Further comments

It may be that this man's presentation with postoperative renal failure was avoidable; if so, use the opportunity to educate your surgical and nursing colleagues.

1.2.20 Diabetic ketoacidosis

Scenario

A 24-year-old student is brought to the Emergency Department by her boyfriend. He tells you that she has been unwell for 3 days and unable to attend lectures. She is a known diabetic and has had difficulty keeping liquids down for 24 hours because she has been vomiting. A fingerprick blood glucose has shown a reading of over 25 mmol/L.

Introduction

⚠ Patients with diabetes, like those with asthma, are used to managing their disease and are often extremely ill by the time they are willing to go to hospital.

History of the presenting problem

Duration of symptoms

How long has she been unwell? Diabetic ketoacidosis (DKA) typically develops over a few days with symptoms including nausea, vomiting, myalgia, headache and abdominal pain.

Evidence of infection

The stress of intercurrent illness is a common cause of loss of diabetic control, interrupted insulin therapy and resultant complications such as DKA. Pursue possible sources of infection: respiratory, urinary, gastrointestinal and skin (ulcers and abscesses) are commonest; septicaemia and meningitis are less likely.

Recent monitoring and management of diabetes

What monitoring of her diabetes has the patient performed over the last few days and what does this reveal? The first common error is for a diabetic to neglect the monitoring of blood glucose when feeling unwell. If monitoring has been performed, this may show evidence of worsening control with progressive hyperglycaemia over the duration of symptom deterioration. The second common error is for the diabetic who is unwell to omit taking any insulin because of inability to eat. Simple poor compliance with insulin therapy can also ultimately result in DKA. Some patients will admit to this, but most often it is information from family or friends or scrutiny of previous accounts in the medical notes that raises this suspicion.

 The two commonest errors of the sick diabetic:

- 'I was feeling too unwell to check my blood sugar.'
- 'I wasn't eating, so I didn't think I needed to take any insulin.'

Other relevant history

Duration and complications of diabetes

It will clearly be necessary to establish the duration of diabetes and whether the patient has suffered

macrovascular complications (eg ischaemic heart disease, cerebrovascular disease and peripheral vascular disease) or microvascular complications (eg neuropathy, nephropathy and retinopathy). Hopefully, she will not have done by the age of 24 years, but if she has had diabetes for 20 years then it is possible.

Usual diabetic control

Previous admissions with DKA or hypoglycaemia would suggest poor diabetic control, poor compliance and lack of education. If there have been previous presentations, is there a pattern to them and is there a common precipitating factor? What has been the HbA$_{1c}$ level?

Examination

The immediate priority, as always, will be to check airway, breathing and circulation (ABC), and determine whether the patient is ill, very ill or nearly dead, with details of further assessment as described in Section 1.2.2. The following would be particularly important aspects in this case.

- Respiratory pattern and breath: does the patient display the sighing respiratory pattern of Kussmaul's breathing induced by acidosis? The smell of ketones on the breath of the patient with DKA may make the diagnosis clear, but not everybody can smell them.

- Assessment of fluid status: patients with DKA are always very volume depleted. In addition to intravascular depletion (postural hypotension, postural tachycardia and low JVP), they are short of interstitial and intracellular fluid (dry mucous membranes, dry axillae, reduced skin turgor and sunken eyes).

- Sources of infection: it is important to consider all sites of potential infection in the diabetic presenting with DKA, especially chest, feet (remove shoes and socks), perianal region and urine (dipstick for nitrites).

- Abdominal: is there abdominal tenderness, silent bowel sounds or pain in the renal angles? Has an intra-abdominal event triggered the DKA? In addition to infection/peritonitis, do not forget bowel infarction, particularly if there is a background of diabetic macrovascular disease. Do not forget a rectal examination: you will not see a perianal abscess unless you look.

> Remember that DKA can mimic an acute abdomen: if in doubt ask for a surgical opinion.

- Neurological: check score on Glasgow Coma Scale to assess this. Also check for the presence of meningeal irritation or focal signs, which would be unlikely but of great significance if present.

There may be signs of chronic damage caused by diabetes (eg retinopathy, neuropathy or vascular disease) but searching for these is not a high priority in the context of the patient presenting with DKA.

Investigation

> DKA is diagnosed by the presence of hyperglycaemia and acidosis, ie low bicarbonate (<15 mmol/L) or low pH (<7.30), with moderate to severe ketonuria.

Urinary ketones
Significant ketonuria, detected by finding a moderately or strongly positive result on Ketostix testing, is

required to establish the diagnosis of DKA.

Routine blood tests

- Blood glucose (laboratory): often the fingerprick blood glucose will read high without a precise value.

- Electrolytes and renal function: serum potassium is likely to be high at presentation, but remember that total body potassium will be significantly depleted. Expect the urea to be elevated out of proportion to the creatinine because of dehydration; compare the creatinine with any previous measurements to determine if renal impairment is acute, chronic or acute on chronic.

- FBC: a raised white cell count might suggest sepsis but can be elevated in the absence of infection in DKA.

- C-reactive protein: to confirm suspicion of sepsis.

- Liver/bone profiles.

Sepsis screen
Send urine for microscopy and culture, blood cultures and other cultures as appropriate, eg sputum and wound swabs. On the CXR look for evidence of infection and also for air under the diaphragm: perforation of an abdominal viscus can be remarkably silent in a diabetic.

Arterial blood gases
DKA produces a metabolic acidosis with respiratory compensation. The presence of ketone bodies from hepatic gluconeogenesis results in a high anion gap, which is calculated as $(Na^+ + K^+) - (Cl^- + HCO_3^-)$, with a normal range of 10–18 mmol/L.

Other investigations
Although it is likely to be normal in this young woman, check an ECG:

myocardial infarction can be a precipitant of DKA and electrolyte disorders can result in arrhythmias. Also perform other imaging tests, eg urinary tract ultrasonography and bone radiographs, as dictated by clinical suspicion.

Management

> **Priorities of management of DKA**
>
> - ABC.
> - Correction of hypovolaemia.
> - Correction of electrolyte imbalance.
> - Correction of hyperglycaemia.
> - Empty the stomach.
> - Treatment of an underlying cause.
> - Prophylaxis against venous thromboembolism.

Fluid resuscitation and electrolyte replacement
Patients with DKA are severely dehydrated and very depleted of total body sodium and potassium: fluid replacement is the top priority. Proceed as described in Section 1.2.2 if hypovolaemic shock is present, but most patients are not profoundly hypotensive and should be given 0.9% (normal) saline with potassium. Typical requirements in the first 24 hours are as shown in Table 10, but the patient will require frequent clinical reassessment over this time and the fluid regimen may need to be adjusted.

> DKA leads to a negative potassium balance because of osmotic diuresis and acidaemia. There will be a rapid decline in serum potassium concentration as it re-enters cells in the first few hours of treatment with rehydration and insulin. Potassium must be replaced as part of the fluid regimen, guided by frequent monitoring of serum potassium throughout treatment.

TABLE 10 FLUID REPLACEMENT IN DKA

Fluid[1]	Volume	Infusion time
0.9% saline	1 L	Over 1 hour
0.9% saline	1 L	Over next 2 hours[2]
0.9% saline	1 L	Over next 4 hours
0.9% saline	1 L	Over next 4 hours
0.9% saline	1 L	Over next 4 hours
0.9% saline	1 L	Over next 4 hours
0.9% saline	1 L	Over next 4 hours

1. When the patient's blood glucose is <10 mmol/L, switch from 0.9% saline to 5% dextrose.
2. After first litre has been administered, add K^+ to infusion solution according to serum K^+ levels, as follows: serum K^+ <3.5 mmol/L, add 40 mmol K^+ to 1 L of infusion solution; serum K^+ 3.5–5.0 mmol/L, add 20 mmol K^+ to 1 L of infusion solution; serum K^+ >5 mmol/L, no addition.

Correction of hyperglycaemia

Insulin therapy reverses ketogenesis, lowers blood glucose and stops the osmotic diuresis. Commence a sliding scale of insulin (Table 11) and monitor blood glucose hourly by the fingerprick method. Note that the insulin infusion should be continued until the serum and urine are clear of ketones and metabolic acidosis has been corrected: this may mean persisting with it after normoglycaemia has been achieved, which can be done if intravenous 5% dextrose replaces 0.9% saline as indicated in Table 10.

Correction of acid–base disturbance

Insulin reverses ketogenesis and causes oxidation of existing ketones, resulting in endogenous bicarbonate production. Restoration of normovolaemia will rapidly reverse the lactate component of metabolic acidosis if there is adequate renal function and tissue perfusion. Treatment with alkali is not routinely required, although administration of bicarbonate should be considered if acidaemia is extreme (pH <7.0) and the patient is hypotensive.

⚠ Bicarbonate administration in DKA should only be considered in extreme acidosis: it may cause exacerbation of hypokalaemia, paradoxical intracellular acidosis due to increased CO_2 production, shift of the oxygen dissociation curve to the left and late alkalosis.

Empty the stomach

Patients with DKA commonly have gastroparesis and several litres of acidic stomach contents waiting to be vomited. Pass a nasogastric tube if the patient is nauseated or vomiting.

Treat infection

Infection is a common precipitant of DKA, particularly pneumonia, urinary tract infection (including pyelonephritis and perinephric abscess), skin sepsis and abscesses. Remember that patients with diabetes may not manifest the classical signs of infection. Have a low threshold for starting empirical broad-spectrum antibiotics after a full septic screen.

Prophylaxis against thromboembolism

An immobile dehydrated patient is at high risk of venous thromboembolism: start low-molecular-weight heparin (prophylactic dose).

Further comments

Cerebral oedema

This is a rare but feared complication of DKA, mostly reported in children or young adults and with a high mortality. Suspect it if the patent complains of a headache or becomes increasingly drowsy and confused. Excessive rehydration and hypertonic fluids can sometimes be responsible. Intensive care unit advice and transfer should be requested urgently if cerebral oedema is suspected.

Hyperosmolar non-ketotic diabetic coma

Hyperosmolar non-ketotic diabetic coma (HONK) must be considered in any case of severe hyperglycaemia. It is typically seen in elderly patients with non-insulin-

TABLE 11 INSULIN SLIDING SCALE FOR THE TREATMENT OF DKA

Blood glucose (mmol/L) measured hourly	Insulin rate (units/hour)
<4	0.5
4.1–7.0	1
7.1–11	2
11.1–15	3
15.1–19	4
19.1–24	5
>24	6

Dilute 50 units of soluble insulin (Actrapid) in 50 mL normal saline and give at the rate indicated (which may need to be adjusted depending on the patient's response).

dependent diabetes and is commonly precipitated by intercurrent illness. Various medications (eg thiazide diuretics and steroids) and consumption of glucose-rich fluids (eg Lucozade) can also precipitate it. Patients are not (by definition) ketoacidotic, but may be acidotic due to lactate accumulation as a result of poor tissue perfusion. The approach to investigation and management is similar to that for DKA, but there are additional points to bear in mind.

Diagnosis Plasma osmolality is calculated as

$$(2 \times Na^+) + (2 \times K^+) + glucose + urea$$

and in HONK is usually >350 mmol/kg. Glucose is usually >40 mmol/L. There may be marked hypernatraemia. Dehydration tends to be severe, causing a disproportionately raised plasma urea. Arterial blood gases are usually relatively normal with pH >7.3 unless there is lactate accumulation.

Treatment The use of hypotonic fluid for rehydration is controversial, the fear being that too rapid reduction of hypernatraemia may result in neurological damage (central pontine myelinolysis) or death. The safest approach is to use 0.9% (normal) saline initially to restore BP and urine flow, and then to change to 0.45% saline if plasma sodium is still >150 mmol/L. Insulin requirements tend to be low, so start at a lower dose of insulin and monitor fingerprick blood glucose closely to avoid hypoglycaemia. Patients with HONK are particularly prone to thromboembolism: anticoagulate with low-molecular-weight heparin as routine.

Why did it happen? Diabetics do not develop DKA or HONK overnight: it builds up over several days. In those known to have diabetes these dangerous conditions are almost invariably avoidable, and when patients have recovered from an episode they should not leave hospital without advice about how to avoid another.

> **Advice to diabetics to prevent DKA or HONK**
>
> - If you get ill, you are likely to need more insulin rather than less.
> - If you get ill, check your blood sugar at least four times a day.
> - If the blood sugar is going up and you do not know what to do, call for help.

1.2.21 Hypoglycaemia

> ### Scenario
>
> A 70-year-old woman with non-insulin-dependent diabetes is brought to the Emergency Department after being found unconscious on the kitchen floor. During transfer to hospital she had a generalised seizure and on arrival she is unresponsive to pain.

Introduction

>
> After checking airway, breathing and circulation (ABC) and then considering opioid toxicity (pinpoint pupils and low respiratory rate), the next priority in dealing with the unconscious patient is measuring fingerprick blood glucose to diagnose or exclude hypoglycaemia (Fig. 32).

The general approach to the unconscious patient is described in Section 1.2.31. This clinical scenario deals with those issues specific to the patient with hypoglycaemia.

History of the presenting problem

> Treat hypoglycaemia first, ask questions afterwards.

Patients in hypoglycaemic coma are not able to give a history. After immediate treatment they may be able to give an account of themselves, but still may not remember key details. Hence ensure that anyone who might know what

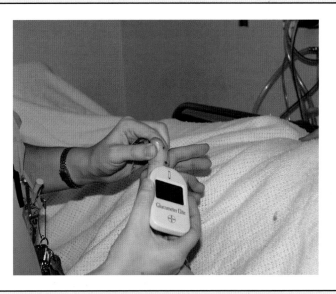

▲ **Fig. 32** Do not ever forget to check a fingerprick blood glucose in a patient who is unconscious.

happened does not disappear from the department while you are treating the patient. Important aspects to ask about include the following.

- History of diabetes: is the patient prone to hypoglycaemia?

- Treatment for diabetes: has this been changed recently?

- Possible precipitating cause, eg alcohol intake or concurrent illness.

- Could the patient have taken an overdose of the medication, either accidental or deliberate?

Examination

As described in Section 1.2.31. Once the patient has responded to treatment, perform a full neurological examination: neurological deficit may persist for days or weeks, and sometimes permanently, despite correction of blood sugar in cases of severe prolonged hypoglycaemia.

Investigation

Hypoglycaemia most commonly arises in known diabetics, who respond rapidly to treatment. Such cases typically require no investigation beyond confirming hypoglycaemia with a fingerprick blood test. In contrast, the hypoglycaemic diabetic who does not respond to glucose requires consideration of other diagnoses, as described in Section 1.2.31.

A much rarer scenario is the patient with hypoglycaemia demonstrated on fingerprick blood test who is not known to be a diabetic. In such cases the differential diagnoses listed in Table 12 should be considered, and blood should be drawn for the following tests before dextrose is given if at all possible (but do not delay treatment while you wait for the results):

- laboratory blood glucose;

- serum to be saved for insulin and C-peptide levels.

Management

> **Urgent treatment is vital if permanent cerebral damage is to be avoided:** any patient with fingerprick blood glucose of <2.5 mmol/L who is unconscious should be given 50 mL of 50% dextrose intravenously immediately.

> ⚠ A patient who is unconscious with a blood glucose of >1.5 mmol/L is unlikely to be unconscious due to hypoglycaemia, but you cannot be completely sure and there can be a terrible penalty for not treating hypoglycaemic coma. If in doubt, treat.

> ⚠ Hypoglycaemia in the 'down-and-out': if there is a history of chronic high alcohol intake or malnourishment, give intravenous thiamine before glucose to avoid precipitating Wernicke's encephalopathy.

If intravenous access is impossible, give 1 mg glucagon im, but remember that this will not work if the hypoglycaemia is due to alcohol.

Note that the half-lives of oral hypoglycaemic agents and medium- and long-acting insulin preparations are both longer than that of glucose. The patient should not be discharged the moment that they become conscious: give a sugary drink and something to eat to prevent recurrent hypoglycaemia, and monitor for at least a few hours (how long will depend on the reason for hypoglycaemia and the social circumstances to which the patient would be discharged). Recheck glucose 15–30 minutes after treatment, and if hypoglycaemia recurs start an infusion of 10% dextrose, aiming to maintain blood glucose at 5–10 mmol/L.

Further comments

Why did it happen?

Hypoglycaemia can strike diabetics out of the blue, but most have some warning. Before patients are discharged, talk through with them what (if anything) they remember of

TABLE 12 CAUSES OF HYPOGLYCAEMIA	
Diabetic patients	**Non-diabetic patients**
Insulin	Concealed insulin administration
Oral hypoglycaemics (especially longer-acting sulphonylureas)	Drugs (eg oral hypoglycaemics, quinine, pentamidine)
Excessive alcohol intake	Salicylate overdose
Excessive exercise	Excessive alcohol (especially chronic alcoholics with liver disease)
	Sepsis
	Insulinoma
	Retroperitoneal sarcoma
	Hypopituitarism
	Adrenocortical insufficiency
	Hypothyroidism
	Liver failure

TABLE 13 CAUSES OF HYPERCALCAEMIA

Cause	Condition
Common	Hyperparathyroidism: primary or tertiary Malignancy: primary or secondary, and especially myeloma Sarcoidosis
Less common/rare	Other granulomatous diseases Excess vitamin D Drugs, particularly thiazide diuretics and lithium Milk/alkali syndrome Other endocrine disorders: thyrotoxicosis, phaeochromocytoma and acute adrenal insufficiency Immobilisation Inappropriate parathyroid hormone (PTH) levels due to altered set point: familial benign hypocalciuric hypercalcaemia

events. Impress upon them that hypoglycaemia is serious: it can be fatal. Tell them that if they get the same feelings again they must check their blood sugar, and that they must have some sugar available to take at all times. With the patient's permission, it is also prudent to offer advice and instruction on how to recognise and handle hypoglycaemia to any of the family and friends that are available.

1.2.22 Hypercalcaemia

> **Scenario**
>
> A 58-year-old man is taken to see his GP by his daughter because he has become increasingly confused and lethargic over the past 5 days. Blood tests are checked, following which the biochemistry department phones the doctor on call for the practice to say that the serum calcium is 3.8 mmol/L (normal range 2.15–2.60). The patient is sent immediately to the Emergency Department where you are asked to review him.

Introduction
Consider the causes of hypercalcaemia, particularly the common ones, as you take the history, examine and investigate (Table 13).

History of the presenting problem
The patient will probably only be able to give a limited history, but ask him and his daughter about symptoms caused by hypercalcaemia. Acute hypercalcaemia can cause fatigue, apathy, anorexia, thirst, polyuria and constipation, with nausea, vomiting, confusion and coma in severe cases. Symptoms of chronic hypercalcaemia include abdominal pain, urinary stones and depression.

Other relevant history
Are there any clues as to the cause of the hypercalcaemia? Consider the diagnoses listed in Table 13 as you enquire about the following.

- Previous history of malignancy.

- Symptoms of malignancy, eg weight loss, back pain, chest or abdominal symptoms, which are usually present when hypercalcaemia is due to cancer.

- Speed of onset of problems: a short history is more typical of hypercalcaemia of malignancy than hypercalcaemia associated with hyperparathyroidism and other diseases.

- Drugs: is the patient receiving thiazide diuretics, vitamin D or lithium?

- Other medications: does the patient have a history of indigestion, and if so is he treating it with over-the-counter remedies or 'white medicine'?

- Is there a concurrent disease predisposing to dehydration or immobility?

> A thorough drug history is essential: patients often do not regard over-the-counter remedies as drugs, particularly ones for a problem as common as indigestion.

Although it seems very likely that this man's confusion is related to his hypercalcaemia, do not forget to consider other possibilities, eg sepsis (could he have pneumonia or a urinary tract infection?), drug side effects (is he on opioids or anything else that might cause confusion?) and other effects of malignancy (eg headache may indicate cerebral metastases).

Examination
Begin with an overall assessment, as described in Section 1.2.2, but key issues will be to assess fluid status, where volume depletion is likely, and look for evidence of malignancy.

Fluid status

- Intravascular volume: check pulse, BP (lying and sitting) and JVP.

- Interstitial/intracellular fluid volume: check skin turgor and mucous membranes.

Evidence of malignancy
The symptoms will point to the type of malignancy.

- General: cachexia, lymphadenopathy and hepatomegaly.

- Lung cancer: clubbing, Horner's syndrome and chest signs.

Clues to other specific causes of confusion and drowsiness

- Check pupils and respiratory rate: small pupils and a low respiratory rate probably mean opioid toxicity. If these features are present, give naloxone as described in Section 1.2.31.

- Look carefully at the fundi: papilloedema suggests raised intracranial pressure. Any clear focal neurological signs would suggest cerebral metastasis in this clinical context.

Investigation

Repeat the measurement of serum calcium to confirm hypercalcaemia; also check electrolytes and renal function (acute renal failure is commonly seen in severe hypercalcaemia), liver/bone profile,

FBC (anaemia may be present for several reasons, most commonly malignant involvement of bone marrow), inflammatory markers, PTH and serum immunoglobulins/ serum protein electrophoresis/ urinary Bence Jones proteins. Perform a CXR, looking in particular for evidence of malignancy (Fig. 33) or features of sarcoidosis.

⚠️ When interpreting serum calcium concentration, remember that free (ionised) plasma calcium is dependent on plasma albumin:

Corrected calcium = measured calcium + {[40 − serum albumin (g/L)] × 0.02}

In most cases the cause of hypercalcaemia will be established by the history, examination and the investigations listed above, but in selected cases the following further tests may be needed: 25-hydroxyvitamin D_3, thyroid function tests, serum angiotensin-converting enzyme, serum magnesium, urinary calcium and creatinine excretion, and bone radiographs.

In any sick patient an ECG should also be performed. In severe hypercalcaemia this can show slowed conduction, including prolonged PR interval, and a widened QRS complex and shortened QT interval with ST segments shortened or absent. Bradyarrhythmias, bundle branch block and atrioventricular block may develop as the serum calcium rises to around 4.5 mmol/L.

Other tests, eg sepsis screen, arterial blood gases and CT brain scan, may be required depending on clinical suspicion.

Management

🔑 **Principles of emergency management of hypercalcaemia**

- Increase urinary excretion of calcium by rehydration with 0.9% saline.
- Inhibit bone resorption with bisphosphonate therapy.

Urgent treatment of hypercalcaemia is needed if there is a reduced consciousness level, confusion, intravascular volume depletion or gross dehydration, or if the patient's serum calcium is more than 3.5 mmol/L (most patients will be symptomatic at this stage).

Rehydration

The first aspect of emergency management should be rehydration with intravenous saline as follows.

- Correct intravascular volume depletion: if this is present (postural tachycardia/hypotension and low JVP), give 0.9% (normal) saline rapidly until the patient is replete (see Section 1.2.2).

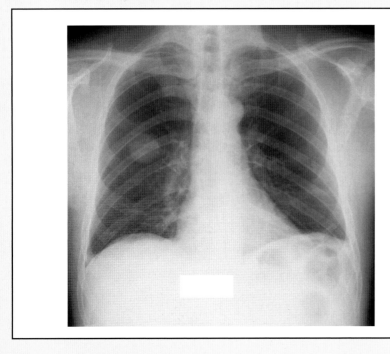

▲**Fig. 33** CXR showing bronchogenic carcinoma.

- When intravascular volume depletion is corrected, give 0.9% (normal) saline intravenously at a rate of around 3–6 L in 24 hours if the patient has a satisfactory urine output. Insert a urinary catheter to monitor urine output. Consider giving furosemide 40–80 mg iv to encourage diuresis. Examine the patient regularly for signs of fluid overload or deficit, ensure accurate fluid charts are kept and adjust fluid input accordingly.

- Monitor the calcium level and also the levels of potassium and magnesium, which may fall rapidly with rehydration. Replace as necessary.

Bisphosphonate therapy

Bisphosphonates are one of the most effective drugs for controlling hypercalcaemia: they bind to hydroxyapatite in calcified bone, which renders it resistant to dissolution, thereby inhibiting both normal and abnormal bone resorption. They have a slow onset of action (1–3 days) but can have a prolonged effect (12–30) days. Disodium pamidronate is the first-choice drug for hypercalcaemia associated with malignancy: 30–90 mg iv is given slowly (over 2–6 hours with 0.5 L of 0.9% saline) into a large vein.

Calcitonin

Calcitonin can be useful in the short-term management of the patient with severe hypercalcaemia: it rapidly (in 2–4 hours) inhibits calcium and phosphorus resorption from the bone and decreases renal calcium reabsorption. The initial dose schedule is 4 units/kg body weight, which is administered subcutaneously or intramuscularly every 12 hours. The dose and schedule may be escalated after 1 or 2 days to 8 units/kg every 12 hours,

and finally to 8 units/kg every 6 hours if the response to lower doses is unsatisfactory. Unfortunately, tachyphylaxis commonly occurs and reduced hypocalcaemic effect is seen with further dosing, indicating that the calcium-lowering effects of calcitonin last for only a few days.

Glucocorticoids

Glucocorticoids are the treatment of choice for hypercalcaemia caused by vitamin D toxicity, sarcoidosis or myeloma. Give hydrocortisone 200 mg iv or prednisolone 40–60 mg orally.

Effect of steroids on hypercalcaemia

The main mechanism of action of steroids is to decrease 1,25-dihydroxyvitamin D levels by inhibiting inflammatory cell proliferation within granulomatous tissue and haematological malignancies. Although the steroids also decrease intestinal calcium absorption and increase urinary calcium excretion, this occurs relatively slowly.

1.2.23 Hyponatraemia

Scenario

A 70-year-old man is brought to the Emergency Department after being found unconscious on a park bench. He has a history of alcohol abuse and is known to have attended the Emergency Department following a minor head injury 4 weeks ago. He is confused, but is moving all his limbs and trying to get off the trolley. He smells strongly of alcohol. No obvious head injury is apparent and he has no focal neurological signs. His fingerprick blood glucose is 6.9 mmol/L. He has routine bloods taken and is

sent to the Clinical Decision Unit pending results and his progress. The nursing staff bleep you with his electrolyte results: Na$^+$ 110 mmol/L, K$^+$ 3.2 mmol/L and urea 2.0 mmol/L.

Introduction

The general approach to the unconscious patient is described in Section 1.2.31. This clinical scenario deals with those issues specific to the patient with hyponatraemia.

Patients vary in their susceptibility to hyponatraemia. Gradual, chronic lowering of the serum sodium concentration is generally much better tolerated than a rapid acute fall; hence symptoms depend not simply on the sodium concentration but its rate of change. However, patients with mild hyponatraemia (sodium 125–135 mmol/L) are usually asymptomatic; those with moderate hyponatraemia (sodium 115–125 mmol/L) may have nausea, malaise, headache, lethargy, restlessness and disorientation; and those with severe hyponatraemia (sodium <115 mmol/L) may suffer seizure, coma and death.

Critical features of hyponatraemia

- Patients with hyponatraemia have too much water: they are almost never short of sodium.
- Hyponatraemia that has developed slowly is often well tolerated and should be corrected slowly, usually with water restriction alone.
- Hyponatraemia that has developed quickly is relatively rare, often iatrogenic and is much more likely to cause symptoms. If it is symptomatic then rapid correction with hypertonic saline may be required, but correction that is too rapid can be associated with dire neurological consequences.

TABLE 14 CAUSES OF HYPONATRAEMIA

Volume status	Total body water	Total extracellular sodium	Primary problem	Example
Hypovolaemic	Low	Even lower	Renal: urinary Na$^+$ >30 mmol/L	Diuretics Sodium-losing renal disorders Mineralocorticoid deficiency
			Non-renal: urinary Na$^+$ <30 mmol/L	Vomiting Diarrhoea Burns Excessive sweating
Euvolaemic	Normal/slight excess	Reduced/normal		SIADH Glucocorticoid deficiency Hypothyroidism 'Sick cells'
Hypervolaemic	Great excess	Excess	Renal: urinary Na$^+$ >30 mmol/L	Acute/chronic renal failure
			Non-renal: urinary Na$^+$ <30 mmol/L	Cardiac failure Cirrhosis/liver failure Nephrotic syndrome

SIADH, syndrome of inappropriate antidiuretic hormone (see Table 15).

Consider the causes of hyponatraemia (Tables 14 and 15) as you try to work out the cause of the problem.

Note that in all cases the development of hyponatraemia requires fluid replacement with hypotonic fluid (by drinking of water or 5% dextrose infusion).

Cause of severe hyponatraemia

The commonest cause is iatrogenic: postoperative infusion of excessive volumes of 5% dextrose solution. Non-osmotic stimuli for ADH release include haemorrhage, nausea, pain and anaesthesia, all of which can be present immediately after operations, leading to enormously high levels of ADH and an inability to excrete water. If a doctor then prescribes large volumes of 5% dextrose, the consequences can be dire.

History and examination

This man will clearly not be able to give a reliable history. Proceed with history and examination as described in Section 1.2.31, but (referring to Tables 14 and 15)

important issues to consider particularly in this case include the following. Could he have a subdural haematoma? Could he have been vomiting (is there evidence of intravascular volume depletion)? Does he have cirrhosis/liver failure or renal failure (what do the notes from his last attendance reveal)? Has he been on treatment with diuretics?

Investigation

This man's neurological state may simply reflect the fact that he is drunk, but it would be unwise to assume that this is the explanation given his profound hyponatraemia. The standard approach to investigation of the unconscious patient is described in Section 1.2.31, but in this case consider the following.

TABLE 15 CAUSES OF SIADH

Source of ADH	Type of problem	Example
Ectopic ADH production	Malignancy	Small-cell lung cancer
Inappropriate pituitary ADH secretion	Malignancy	Lung cancer, lymphoma, prostate cancer, pancreatic cancer
	Inflammatory lung disease	Pneumonia, lung abscess
	Neurological disease	Meningitis, head injury, subdural haematoma, tumours, post surgery
	Drugs	Antidepressants (tricyclics and SSRIs), carbamazepine, chlorpropamide, phenothiazines (eg chlorpromazine), vincristine, cyclophosphamide, ecstasy
	Postoperative[1]	–
	Others	Nausea, pain, porphyria

1. See Hazard box to the left of this table.
ADH, antidiuretic hormone; SSRIs, selective serotonin reuptake inhibitors.

CT brain scan

It would be appropriate to image the brain even in the absence of focal neurological signs given that this man is an alcoholic with a history of recent head injury and that subdural haematoma can be associated with SIADH.

Cause of hyponatraemia

Urinary sodium concentration (urine 'spot sodium') is useful for distinguishing between renal and extrarenal hypovolaemic hyponatraemia, as well as between causes of hypervolaemic hyponatraemia (see Table 14). Paired urine and plasma osmolalities should be sent along with the spot sodium: measurement of these is required to pursue the possibility of SIADH. Remember, however, that this is a diagnosis of exclusion and not proven simply by finding that the urine is hypotonic. Further investigations will depend on the underlying suspected cause.

> **The following criteria for the diagnosis of SIADH must all be satisfied to confirm the dignosis:**
>
> - plasma osmolality <270 mosmol/kg with inappropriate urinary concentration (>100 mosmol/kg);
> - patient is euvolaemic and not taking a diuretic;
> - renal sodium excretion >20 mmol/L;
> - normal renal, thyroid and adrenal function.

Management

The correct strategy for management of hyponatraemia depends on whether the patient is symptomatic as a result of it. Harm can be done by overzealous correction: in the case of an elderly woman who is relatively well but hyponatraemic due to diuretic treatment, she is much more likely to suffer than to benefit from an aggressive medical

approach. This man is a difficult case: he is probably symptomatic as a result of severe acute hyponatraemia and I would treat him as such, while remaining alert to the fact that there could be other reasons for his mental state.

Asymptomatic hyponatraemia

Management of the patient with asymptomatic hyponatraemia depends on identifying and treating (where possible) the underlying cause (Table 14), coupled with restriction of fluid input to 1 L/day to enable the serum sodium concentration to rise. Such fluid restriction can be difficult for patients to tolerate and for nurses to enforce: give the allocation in aliquots throughout the day; give it as ice cubes to suck; and permit the patient swabs to keep the mouth moist or to suck boiled sweets.

>
>
> **Hyponatraemia alone will very rarely cause neurological symptoms when the concentration is <120 mmol/L. If the serum sodium concentration is higher than this in a comatose patient, consider other causes of coma.**

Symptomatic hyponatraemia

Urgent treatment is required if there are severe neurological effects, eg fitting. Aside from treating the underlying cause, use hypertonic saline to elevate the patient's serum sodium concentration. However, remember that central pontine myelinolysis is reported in association with over-rapid correction and note the following.

- No formula can accurately predict the patient's response to hypertonic saline. All formulae assume a 'closed system' and take no account of the patient's

ongoing water losses, which are not predicatable.

- 1.8% saline infused at a rate of (1.7 × patient's weight in kg) mL/hour or 3% saline infused at a rate of (1.0 × patient's weight in kg) mL/hour is likely to increase the serum sodium concentration by 1 mmol/L per hour.

- Aim to increase the serum sodium concentration in the early stages of correction by about 1 mmol/L per hour and by no more than 15–20 mmol/L over 48 hours.

- Monitor the serum sodium concentration every 2 hours while infusing hypertonic saline, and replace hypertonic saline with 0.9% saline if the serum sodium is rising more quickly than desired.

- Stop the infusion of hypertonic saline when serum sodium is >125 mmol/L and institute water restriction: do not allow rapid correction into the normal range.

> **⚠ Treatment of severe hyponatraemia**
>
> Correction of symptomatic hyponatraemia with hypertonic saline requires very close monitoring: check serum sodium every 2 hours.

1.2.24 Addisonian crisis

Scenario

A 32-year-old woman is brought to the Emergency Department by her husband. He explains that she collapsed today at work and was sent home. She has been unwell for some time with lethargy and dizziness, and has lost a significant amount of weight. On arrival she is drowsy, confused and complaining of abdominal pain. She looks unwell and has BP 80/50 mmHg. Urgent bloods are taken by the physician's assistant. You are in the process of assessing her when the biochemistry results become available, showing Na⁺ 128 mmol/L and K⁺ 5.8 mmol/L.

Introduction

The clinical approach to the patient with hypotension is discussed in Section 1.2.2, but in this case there are a number of clues that this is an acute-on-chronic presentation: the patient has been unwell for some time suggesting a chronic disease process, and there are clear clues to acute adrenal insufficiency (addisonian crisis), ie hypotension with mild hyponatraemia and hyperkalaemia.

History of the presenting problem

A thorough history is obviously required, but the information available means that you should enquire carefully about features that would support the diagnosis of adrenal insufficiency.

Features suggesting chronic adrenal insufficiency

Non-specific symptoms are a dominant feature: dizziness on standing caused by postural hypotension is common, many patients report constipation or diarrhoea, and progressive weight loss can be an important clue to the insidious development of the disease. If asked directly many patients will report a craving for salt.

Features suggesting addisonian crisis

About 25% of patients with Addison's disease present in crisis, with rapid progression of their symptoms. Many cases develop non-specific abdominal pain in conjunction with nausea and/or vomiting, and also restlessness and confusion, which in some patients can progress to stupor and coma.

Is there any history to suggest an underlying precipitant of the crisis?

Any intercurrent illness may precipitate an addisonian crisis, when in rare cases a history of flank pain may be due to haemorrhagic adrenal infarction.

Other relevant history

Drug history

Previous steroid usage may have caused adrenal suppression and left the patient vulnerable to an addisonian crisis in the event of intercurrent illness. Rifampicin and ketoconazole can also cause primary hypoadrenalism in some patients.

> Patients on long-term steroids require additional steroids to cover intercurrent illness/stress.

Autoimmune diseases

In the UK autoimmune disease accounts for about 80% of cases of Addison's disease, in whom it is associated with other autoimmune conditions including vitiligo, pernicious anaemia, thyroiditis, type 1 diabetes mellitus and hypoparathyroidism.

Other possible underlying causes

Tuberculosis (TB) and malignancy can cause adrenal failure.

Examination

Resuscitation as described in Section 1.2.2 will be the immediate priority, but in view of the suspicion of Addison's disease in this case you should, aside from concentrating on the state of the circulation and looking for evidence of sepsis as a precipitant of crisis, look carefully for pigmentation (Fig. 34) and also for vitiligo.

Given the presentation with abdominal pain it will clearly be important to check carefully for signs of intra-abdominal mischief.

Investigation

The approach to investigation of the very ill patient is described in Section 1.2.2, but in this case particularly consider the following.

Routine investigation of the ill patient

Blood glucose may be low, with symptomatic hypoglycaemia. Electrolytes/renal function tests classically show hyponatraemia, hyperkalaemia (as in this case) and a high urea, but they can be normal. Hypercalcaemia can be seen in conjunction with significant dehydration, but is sometimes seen after rehydration. FBC may show anaemia, or a raised white cell count if there is an infective precipitant. The CXR is likely to show a small heart and may show pneumonia as a precipitant of crisis. Adrenal calcification from old TB may be visible on an abdominal radiograph.

> The typical findings in acute adrenal insufficiency are hyponatraemia, hyperkalaemia and hypoglycaemia.

Establishing the diagnosis of adrenal insufficiency

- Random cortisol measurement: if possible take a sample before administration of steroid, but remember that random cortisol measurements are difficult to

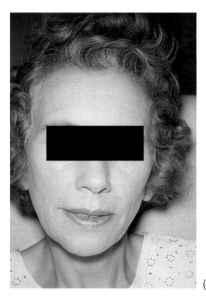

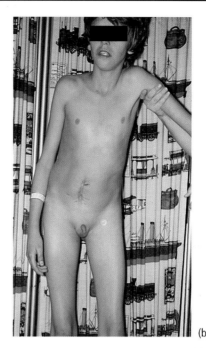

(a)

(b)

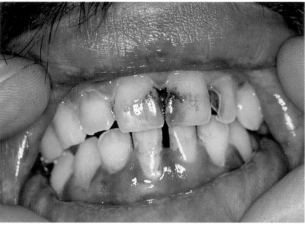

(c)

▲ **Fig. 34** Hyperpigmentation of the skin (**a, b**) and buccal tissues (**c**) in patients with Addison's disease.

interpret and should be viewed with caution.

- Short adrenocorticotrophic hormone (ACTH; Synacthen) stimulation test: in this case it would be dangerous and wrong to delay treatment, but in less dramatic circumstances this should be a priority if adrenal insufficiency is suspected. Synacthen 0.25 mg im/iv is administered to the patient (time 0); samples for measurement of plasma cortisol are collected at 0, +30 and +60 minutes; a cortisol level >550 nmol/L (with rise from baseline >190 nmol/L) excludes

the diagnosis of primary adrenal failure.

- Plasma ACTH: a high level (>80 ng/L) with low or low-normal cortisol confirms primary hypoadrenalism.

It will be appropriate to check thyroid function in all cases of adrenal insufficiency. If hydrocortisone is given acutely, as should be done in this case, then short (or long) Synacthen testing can be done at a later date after the omission of hydrocortisone for 24 hours or substitution with dexamethasone. Further

endocrinological investigations, eg pituitary function tests, will be required in selected cases.

Management

Key aspects of resuscitation in this case include the following.

- Fluids: the patient in addisonian crisis is significantly depleted of both salt and water. Aggressive fluid resuscitation with 0.9% saline is vital.

- Glucocorticoid replacement: give hydrocortisone 100–200 mg iv immediately, and then 100 mg iv three times daily. Fludrocortisone replacement will need to be considered in the long term, but in the acute situation hydrocortisone is the treatment of choice.

- Beware the risk of hypoglycaemia: monitor fingerprick blood glucose regularly. Start a 10% dextrose drip if necessary and run it at a rate to keep glucose >5 mmol/L, but do not give more than is needed and avoid using 5% dextrose because it is more likely to exacerbate hyponatraemia.

- Consider sepsis: have a low threshold for treating with empirical antibiotics.

Shoot first, ask questions afterwards

Give steroids immediately if you suspect addisonian crisis.

1.2.25 Thyrotoxic crisis

Scenario

A 45-year-old woman is brought to the Emergency Department because she has become increasingly paranoid over the past few days. She is known to have 'a thyroid problem' but has recently become interested in homeopathic medicine and stopped taking her usual tablets. She is also agitated and delusional so taking a history is not straightforward, but she has clearly lost a lot of weight, has a marked tremor, is febrile and is tachycardic. You are asked to assess her urgently by the nurse in charge.

History of the presenting problem

Getting a detailed history is not possible in this case, but the problem

is clear-cut: features of a thyrotoxic crisis (storm) include weight loss, heat intolerance, sweating, palpitations, diarrhoea, tremor and anxiety/agitation/irritability.

Possible precipitating causes of a thyrotoxic crisis include withdrawal of antithyroid drug therapy (as in this case), but also infection, radioiodine treatment, iodinated contrast dyes, thyroid surgery and childbirth.

Examination

The approach to the examination of the very ill patient is described in Section 1.2.2, but in this case you would obviously look for features that would be consistent with a diagnosis of thyrotoxic crisis.

- General: agitation, anxiety and restlessness; tremor; the skin is usually warm and moist; and hyperpyrexia, a feature of thyrotoxic crisis that does not necessarily indicate infection, although this should always be looked for.

- Cardiovascular compromise: sinus tachycardia is usually greater than 140 bpm in thyroid crisis (storm); fast atrial fibrillation or supraventricular tachycardia is common. Is there cardiac failure: raised JVP, gallop rhythm, pulmonary oedema and peripheral oedema?

- Neurological/psychological: altered consciousness, frank psychosis, delirium, seizures and coma can all be seen in thyrotoxic crisis.

Findings that might indicate the likely cause of the thyroid pathology include the following.

- Signs of Graves' disease (Fig. 35): exophthalmos, lid retraction and lid lag.

- Is there a goitre? If so, what are its characteristics (smooth, nodular or painful) and is there an associated bruit?

- Vitiligo: associated with autoimmune thyroid disease.

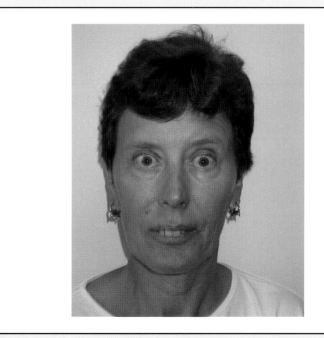

▲**Fig. 35** A patient with exophthalmos and lid retraction due to Graves' disease.

Investigation

> **Thyrotoxic crisis is a clinical diagnosis**
>
> There are no laboratory criteria to diagnose thyrotoxic crisis: the levels of thyroid hormones are the same as in uncomplicated hyperthyroidism. Start treatment immediately if the clinical diagnosis is thyrotoxic crisis. Do not delay while waiting for laboratory confirmation.

The approach to investigation of the very ill patient is described in Section 1.2.2, but in this case the following would be particularly important.

- ECG: sinus tachycardia is expected, but look for atrial fibrillation or other arrhythmia.

- Thyroid function tests: clear evidence of hyperthyroidism would be expected, but in this clinical context you should not wait for confirmation before beginning treatment.

Management

Thyrotoxic crisis is a life-threatening condition, with mortality of up to 20–30% reported. Aside from basic resuscitation (see Section 1.2.2), give specific treatment for thyrotoxic crisis on clinical suspicion.

Hyperthyroidism

The patient in thyrotoxic crisis requires both of the following.

- Propylthiouracil or carbimazole: propylthiouracil is the preferred drug as it both blocks further synthesis of thyroid hormones and inhibits peripheral conversion of T_4 to T_3. However, it is often not immediately available on the wards, whereas carbimazole usually is. If propylthiouracil is

available, give a loading dose of 600 mg to 1 g orally or via a nasogastric tube, then 200 mg every 6 hours. If propylthiouracil is not available (you should not wait for the pharmacy to 'get some up to the ward tomorrow'), give carbimazole 20 mg, then 20 mg three times daily.

- Lugol's iodine (saturated solution of potassium iodide): five drops every 5 hours, beginning 4 hours after starting propylthiouracil/ carbimazole (not before, as thyroid hormone stores may be increased) to inhibit further release of thyroxine.

Supportive measures particular to thyrotoxic crisis

- Hyperpyrexia: peripheral cooling measures and paracetamol. Do not use aspirin as it can displace thyroid hormone from its binding sites.

- Tachycardia: give propranolol 1 mg iv, repeated every 20 minutes as necessary up to total of 5 mg, or give 40–80 mg po four times daily. Be careful if the patient has cardiac failure. Esmolol, a short-acting beta-blocker, can be used as an infusion for immediate management of sympathetic overactivity.

- Atrial fibrillation: consider digitalisation, but note that higher doses of digoxin than usual may be needed due to relative resistance to the drug.

- Steroids: hydrocortisone 200 mg iv, then 100 mg every 6 hours; or dexamethasone 2 mg po four times daily.

Treat possible precipitating causes

Start broad-spectrum antibiotics if there is any suggestion of infection.

1.2.26 Sudden onset of severe headache

Scenario

A 34-year-old woman presents to the Emergency Department with sudden onset of severe occipital headache. You are the duty medical doctor on call and are asked to assess her.

Introduction

> 🔑 Sudden-onset severe headache is due to subarachnoid haemorrhage until proved otherwise.

History of the presenting problem

Features of the headache to enquire about include the following.

- Speed of onset: subarachnoid haemorrhage (SAH) comes on suddenly.

- Severity: patients usually describe the pain of SAH as the worst they have ever had, and often 'like being hit over the head with a baseball bat'.

- Time of onset: headaches that wake the patient from sleep (rather than being noticed on waking) are significant, as are those occurring on exercise, including sexual activity.

Have there been any other symptoms such as nausea, vomiting, blurring of vision or any other neurological dysfunction, and did these come on before or after the headache? Did the patient lose consciousness for any period? Migraine is often associated with a visual aura prior to the onset of headache; SAH may give negative symptoms such as loss of consciousness, visual impairment or weakness that follow the headache. Photophobia is a feature of SAH, but also of meningitis and migraine.

Other relevant history

Has the patient had headaches in the past and if so were they like this? If patients with a history of headache do have SAH, they almost always identify the pain as being different. Does the patient smoke or use illicit drugs (amphetamine and cocaine are associated with SAH, as is smoking)? Ask about any family history of SAH or related conditions (adult polycystic kidney disease and some connective tissue diseases).

Are there features to support another diagnosis? Have there been any recent problems with the eyes, ears or sinuses that could indicate sinusitis or otitis media? Has the patient travelled abroad recently or had symptoms to suggest infection? Could this be meningitis or malaria (see Section 1.2.27)?

Examination

Patients with severe headache range from those who walk into the Emergency Department to those who are comatose with cardiorespiratory collapse. The general approach to the examination of the patient in coma is discussed in Section 1.2.31, and for the patient with cardiovascular collapse in Section 1.2.2. In dealing with the patient with suspected SAH, aside from assessing and alleviating pain and anxiety, the following are of particular importance.

- Check score on Glasgow Coma Scale (Fig. 40) immediately to establish baseline.

- Focal neurological signs, especially pupillary size and reaction: a fixed dilated pupil is an extremely worrying physical sign

in this context, indicating damage to the third cranial nerve either from generalised compression (raised intracranial pressure) or localised compression (aneurysm of the posterior communicating artery).

- Features of SAH: neck stiffness, subconjunctival haemorrhages (also a feature of meningococcal disease, but subconjunctival haemorrhages where you cannot see the lateral limits are indicative of SAH) and subhyaloid haemorrhages. Also check for features (much less likely) of connective tissue diseases and for adult polycystic kidney disease, which predispose to SAH.

- Features to support another diagnosis: high fever; and infection of ears, nose and throat.

Investigation

The general approach to investigation of the patient in coma is discussed in Section 1.2.31. With regard to general investigations, note that SAH is often associated with cardiac dysfunction.

- ECG shows ST- and T-wave changes in 70–80% of cases, including an infarct pattern in 10–15%.

- CXR shows either neurogenic or cardiogenic pulmonary oedema developing in 10–15% of patients.

- Serum troponin level is often slightly or moderately elevated.

CT brain scan

About 90% of SAHs are visible on a CT scan (Fig. 36), which is the investigation of choice. Patients who present some days after onset of symptoms may be difficult to diagnose as the degradation of blood means that it may have the same density as brain tissue.

Lumbar puncture

All patients suspected of having an SAH but with a negative CT scan should be considered for lumbar puncture if there are no contraindications (see Section 3.2). This should be performed a minimum of 12 hours after the onset of symptoms; before this time breakdown products of red cells in

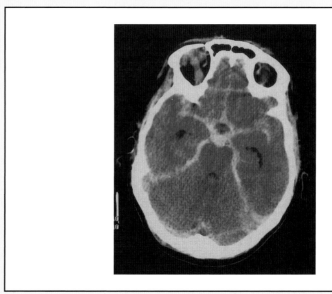

▲**Fig. 36** Unenhanced CT scan showing blood outlining the circle of Willis in a patient with SAH.

the cerebrospinal fluid (CSF) may not be apparent. At least three serial CSF specimens should be examined for xanthochromia and red cell count.

> ⚠ In suspected SAH wait 12 hours from the onset of symptoms before performing lumbar puncture to avoid a false-negative result.

Management

The important features of medical management of aneurysmal SAH are as follows.

- Analgesia: SAH is described as being the most severe pain imaginable. Pain will increase the catecholamine response, potentially increasing the risk of rebleeding or cardiac dysfunction.

- Oxygen: all patients should receive high-flow oxygen. There will be a penumbral area around the region of the SAH that is at risk of ischaemic damage.

- Fluid: assuming they have normal renal function and adequate urinary output, patients should receive at least 3 L/day of 0.9% saline. Solutions containing dextrose should be avoided: once the dextrose is consumed, the fluid is hypotonic and will preferentially move into cerebral cells, thereby worsening cerebral oedema.

- Nimodipine: a selective calcium channel blocker that preferentially acts on the cerebral microcirculation to reduce the risk of vasospasm. Nimodipine 60 mg po every 4 hours for 3 weeks should be given to all patients with SAH who are not hypotensive (systolic BP <110 mmHg).

- Bed-rest, and aperients to avoid excessive straining when opening the bowels.

> 🔑 All patients with SAH should be discussed with the regional neurosurgical centre unless they are terminally ill for some other reason.

Further comments

Major intracerebral complications of SAH

- Rebleeding: the risk of rebleeding from a cerebral aneurysm following acute SAH is about 4% in the first 24 hours and 1% per day thereafter.

- Hydrocephalus: the risk depends on both the volume and site of blood within the subarachnoid space. Large bleeds are more likely to cause hydrocephalus through blockage of the arachnoid granulations responsible for reabsorption of CSF: blood clots situated in narrow areas of the ventricular system, such as the third ventricle or the aqueduct, may cause obstructive hydrocephalus.

- Vasospasm (delayed ischaemic neurological deficit): generally occurs 5–12 days after SAH. Breakdown products of blood are thought to trigger vasospasm of nearby arteries, resulting in symptomatic ischaemia that may be irreversible.

Definitive treatments for aneurysmal SAH

- Clipping: the patient requires a general anaesthetic and craniotomy, when a surgical clip is placed around the neck of the aneurysm.

- Coiling: the patient requires a general anaesthetic. A catheter is inserted, usually via a femoral artery, and manoeuvred to the site of the aneurysm; thrombogenic coils are placed within the aneurysm to secure it.

If both techniques are available in a given centre, the decision regarding coiling versus clipping depends on the site and nature of the aneurysm, the number of aneurysms present and the comorbidity of the patient.

1.2.27 Severe headache with fever

> ### Scenario
>
> A 22-year-old student presents with 24 hours of increasing headache associated with high fever and a rash. Previously he was well. You are the on-call medical doctor and are asked to see him in the Emergency Department.

Introduction

> 🔑 This man almost certainly has meningococcal meningitis and must be treated as such immediately.

History of the presenting problem

> 🔑 Before embarking on taking a history the top priority is to determine if the patient is well, ill, very ill or nearly dead. If the latter, get help from the intensive care unit immediately.

If circumstances permit history-taking, then ask about the following.

- Onset of headache: the headache of meningitis is usually a dull, progressively worsening one, in contrast to that of subarachnoid haemorrhage (see Section 1.2.26).

- Systemic features: 'flu-like symptoms of fever, sweats, muscle aches, joint pains and nausea/vomiting suggest systemic infection and are common in meningitis.

- Photophobia: a common complaint in meningitis but also seen with migraine and subarachnoid haemorrhage. Do not over-interpret this symptom: anyone with a severe headache of any cause will be averse to bright lights.

- Sore throat and earache: these may be the primary cause of the headache or may indicate the source of meningitis.

- Behaviour: recent changes in behaviour might point towards meningoencephalitis.

Other relevant history

Given the immediate working diagnosis of meningococcal meningitis, has the patient been in contact with anyone with meningitis? Where does he live, who are his close contacts and have any of these been ill recently? Contacts will need to be traced and appropriate antibiotic prophylaxis given if the case is confirmed as due to meningococcal disease.

It will also be important to ask about whether the patient has received any antibiotics recently, which may prevent successful culture of the organism, and if they have any allergies especially to penicillin.

Examination

The general approach to the examination of the patient in coma is discussed in Section 1.2.31, and for the patient with cardiovascular collapse in Section 1.2.2. In dealing with a case of suspected meningococcal meningitis, note the following.

Skin, mucous membranes and eyes

Any new rash should be treated as highly suspicious. Although the rash of meningococcal septicaemia is classically purplish and non-blanching (Fig. 37), in its early stages it may be erythematous and macular. Look for infarcts in the nail-beds, resulting from immune complex deposition. Look carefully for subconjunctival and sublingual haemorrhages. Look in the fundi for subhyaloid haemorrhages and papilloedema.

Features of meningeal irritation

Several physical signs are described, the most common being the following.

- Neck stiffness: there is involuntary resistance to flexion when the physician attempts to bend the patient's neck such that the chin touches the chest. The best known of several signs attributed to Brudzinski is positive when such flexion of the patient's neck causes flexion of both hips and knees.

- Kernig's sign: the patient lies in bed with hip and knee flexed; a positive sign is recorded when an attempt by the physician to extend the knee is resisted involuntarily by the patient (and usually causes pain).

Investigation

 Suspected meningococcal septicaemia

Treat first, ask questions afterwards.

The general approaches to investigation of the patient who is very ill or in coma are discussed in Sections 1.2.2 and 1.2.31. In this case the particular emphasis will clearly be on trying to confirm the diagnosis of meningococcal septicaemia/meningitis.

Insert an intravenous cannula, draw blood cultures through it and give intravenous antibiotics.

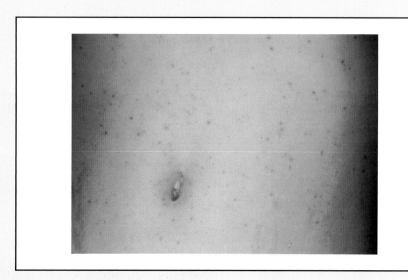

▲**Fig. 37** Characteristic petechial rash of meningococcal septicaemia.

Neisseria meningitidis can be cultured from blood, scrapings of skin lesions and cerebrospinal fluid; the diagnosis of meningococcal disease may also be made immunologically. See Section 3.2 for discussion of contraindications, technique and interpretation of the findings of lumbar puncture.

Management

Aside from supportive care, described in Section 1.2.2, the essential requirement is to give an appropriate antibiotic without delay. The choice depends on local sensitivities, but is usually a high-dose cephalosporin, eg cefotaxime 2 g iv every 4 hours or ceftriaxone 2 g iv every 12 hours.

Further comments

Meningitis is a notifiable disease: refer the case to public health for contact tracing. Household and other intimate contacts are recommended to take prophylactic antibiotics (eg a single dose of ciprofloxacin 750 mg orally) and to be immunised (if meningococcaemia is due to serogroup C or A).

1.2.28 Acute spastic paraparesis

Scenario

A 38-year-old woman is referred urgently by her GP. For the last 3 days she has had mild bilateral leg weakness with difficulty climbing stairs. She has not passed urine for 18 hours and is distressed. You are asked to see and assess her.

Introduction

The diagnosis in this case is cord compression until proved otherwise, but consider the possibilities listed in Table 16 as you deal with the case.

TABLE 16 CAUSES OF ACUTE OR SUBACUTE PARAPLEGIA OR QUADRIPLEGIA

Frequency	General type of cause	Clinical condition
Common	Cord compression	Primary/secondary tumour Herniated disc
	Other	Guillain–Barré syndrome Transverse myelitis (idiopathic, MS, SLE, Behçet's syndrome, HIV)
Must consider	Vascular causes	Aortic dissection Spinal cord SAH Thrombosis of anterior spinal artery
	Cord compression	Epidural abscess Osteomyelitis (including TB)
	Other	Deficiency diseases (B_{12} deficiency, beriberi, alcoholic neuropathy)
Rare		Toxic polyneuropathies Severe hypokalaemia Tick paralysis Porphyric polyneuropathy

MS, multiple sclerosis; SAH, subarachnoid haemorrhage; SLE, systemic lupus erythematosus; TB, tuberculosis.

History of the presenting problem

Important aspects to explore include the following.

- Speed of progression: cord compression is usually acute, producing non-progressive and asymmetric weakness. Guillain–Barré syndrome typically presents as a distal weakness, usually with tingling or a tight 'bound' sensation of the distal lower limbs, and progresses steadily over a few days.

- Presence or absence of pain: sudden onset of pain in association with weakness suggests a herniated disc, spinal subarachnoid haemorrhage or aortic dissection with involvement of the spinal arteries.

- Sensory symptoms: these (usually painful) often precede weakness by some days or even weeks in cord compression; in Guillain–Barré syndrome they usually occur simultaneously or slightly later.

- Bladder or bowel involvement: urinary or bowel dysfunction suggests cord compression.

- Associated symptoms: anorexia, malaise and weight loss should raise the possibility of disseminated malignancy. Fever, rigors or sweats suggest osteomyelitis, TB or an epidural abscess.

> ⚠ Breathlessness in the patient with paraparesis or quadriparesis is a sinister symptom: respiratory failure can be rapidly progressive in Guillain–Barré syndrome and around one-third of patients require ventilatory support.

Other relevant history

A thorough past medical history is crucial: is there any previous history of malignancy, eg breast cancer, or of a multisystem disorder such as SLE? Previous neurological symptoms might point to a diagnosis of MS. Intravenous drug usage may lead to osteomyelitis, epidural abscess or (less likely) transverse myelitis in association with HIV infection.

Examination: general features

Poor general health may indicate malignancy, anorexia or nutritional deficiencies. Breast and thyroid examination are important to exclude two malignancies that can metastasise to the spine in this age group.

Cardiovascular abnormalities, eg tachycardia, bradycardia, hypertension or hypotension, may indicate autonomic dysfunction in association with Guillain–Barré syndrome.

Respiratory assessment is especially important in suspected Guillain–Barré syndrome. Can the patient speak in full sentences or only words at a time? A simple method to quantitate respiratory disability is to ask the patient to take a deep breath and then to count out loud as far as possible (1, 2, 3, 4 . . .). This correlates fairly well with forced vital capacity and can be easily reproduced to assess if things are getting better or worse.

Is the patient's bladder palpable? Autonomic involvement may occur in a variety of conditions, including Guillain–Barré syndrome, but the most urgent need is to exclude cord compression.

Examination: nervous system

Evidence of cord compression

- Motor: below the level of an acute cord compression, weakness may be associated with hypotonia, hyporeflexia and unresponsive plantars, although hypertonia, hyperreflexia and upgoing plantars develop rapidly and will be found at presentation in many cases.

- Sensory: examine carefully for a sensory level, possibly suspended, that defines the most caudal location of a spinal lesion that could be responsible for the patient's symptoms and signs. Do not forget to check sensation in the saddle area, impairment suggesting a lesion in the cauda equina.

The finding of neurological signs above the level of a cord lesion clearly indicates that more than one neurological site is affected, eg optic atrophy in a patient with MS, or cerebral and spinal metastases in a patient with disseminated malignancy.

> ⚠️ **Urinary retention is not always due to mechanical outflow obstruction**
>
> When performing a rectal examination in a patient with urinary retention, always ask 'Can you feel me touching you here?' before you start. Patients with cord compression can present with urinary retention and little in the way of leg weakness.

> 🔑 Sphincter disturbance, sensory loss in the saddle area and ankle weakness suggests a cauda equina lesion.

Evidence of Guillain–Barré syndrome

- Motor: lower motor neuron weakness, distal more than proximal, with reduced tone and areflexia. Facial involvement and ophthalmoplegia is found in the Miller Fisher syndrome variant.

- Sensory: glove and stocking sensory loss, which is often mild.

Investigation

> 🔑 Investigation and treatment of spinal cord compression is an emergency. Incomplete lesions with sparing of part of the sensory or motor pathways have a much better prognosis than complete lesions: rarely can function be restored once lost. Discuss lesions immediately with radiological colleagues and neurosurgical services.

Imaging of the spine

MRI is the investigation of choice in patients with non-traumatic paraplegia or quadriplegia (Fig. 38). Plain radiography of the spine may show an obvious lesion. A CT scan or a myelogram may be indicated in individual patients, although CT scanning may not exclude cord compression and may not show

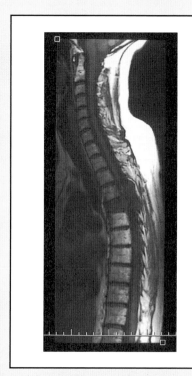

▲ **Fig. 38** MRI (T2-weighted image) showing a spinal secondary deposit causing cord compression.

evidence of demyelination, and myelography can cause clinical deterioration in patients with cord compression.

Other tests

Routine haematological and biochemical screening tests will be required, with particular emphasis on looking for evidence of malignancy (anaemia, abnormal liver blood tests, hypercalcaemia, raised inflammatory markers and abnormalities on CXR) and, in an older patient, myeloma (serum immunoglobulins, serum protein electrophoresis and urinary Bence Jones proteinuria). Other investigations may be appropriate depending on the clinical context, eg cultures to pursue sepsis/TB and lymph node biopsy.

If Guillain–Barré syndrome is a possibility

This is primarily a clinical diagnosis but can be supported by lumbar puncture (after cord compression excluded by imaging; typically reveals elevated protein with normal cell count), nerve conduction studies (absence or impersistence of F waves) and anti-GQ1b antibodies (positive in Miller Fisher variant). Check stool culture and serology for *Campylobacter jejuni*, serology for atypical pneumonia and cerebrospinal fluid for viral infection.

Because of concern about respiratory or cardiac involvement, check and continue to monitor respiratory function tests (forced expiratory volume in 1 second), arterial blood gases and ECG.

Management

Specific treatments will depend on the diagnosis, but the following are important for all patients with acute paraplegia:

- relieve urinary retention (if present);
- give adequate analgesia;
- provide a pressure-relieving mattress and turn the patient over regularly to prevent pressure sores;
- early institution of bowel care.

Cord compression

Disc protrusion requires surgical decompression. Metastatic disease may be treated with high-dose steroids followed by surgical decompression or radiotherapy, depending on the context. Spinal/epidural abscess requires surgical drainage and appropriate antimicrobials.

Guillain–Barré syndrome

Give intravenous immunoglobulin 0.4 g/kg daily for 5 days. Antiarrhythmic and antihypertensive drugs may be required, but use them with caution and obtain expert help in dealing with these problems that can arise with autonomic instability.

1.2.29 Status epilepticus

Scenario

A man who seems to be about 50 years old has been found collapsed in the street with generalised seizures. He has been fitting continuously for 20 minutes by the time he reaches the Emergency Department. No past history is available and no family members or friends are present.

Immediate management

- Assess airway, breathing and circulation, and initiate resuscitation if required (see Sections 1.2.1 and 1.2.2).

- Give high-flow oxygen; apply a pulse oximeter to monitor oxygen saturation.
- Obtain intravenous access.
- Check fingerprick blood glucose; if <2.5 mmol/L, give 50 mL of 50% dextrose intravenously. Also give high-potency thiamine (eg Pabrinex or Parenterovite) to patients with poor nutrition.

⚠️ Insertion of an oral airway is almost impossible during a fit and is likely to cause trauma to either the teeth or the soft tissues if performed: wait until the fit has terminated and then insert an oral or nasal airway as necessary.

🔑 To terminate status epilepticus give either lorazepam or diazepam.

- Lorazepam (4 mg iv at a rate of 2 mg/min): watch for sedation, respiratory depression and hypotension. This terminates fits in 60–90% of patients.
- Diazepam (10–20 mg iv at a rate of 5 mg/min): can be given rectally at a dose of 10–20 mg (rectal gel) if intravenous access cannot be obtained.

Also give fosphenytoin or phenytoin.

- Fosphenytoin (15–20 mg phenytoin equivalents/kg iv at a rate of 150 mg/min): 50% of patients who have not responded to the initial benzodiazepine will do so with the addition of fosphenytoin.
- Phenytoin (15–20 mg/kg iv at a rate of 25–50 mg/min).

Call for anaesthetic help if there is still no response: the patient may need to be fully anaesthetised using barbiturates or non-barbiturate drugs (eg propofol), intubated and ventilated.

TABLE 17 CAUSES OF STATUS EPILEPTICUS	
Common	**Must consider**
Primary epilepsy	Space-occupying lesion
Hypoglycaemia	Anoxia
SAH/CVA	Intracerebral infection and meningitis
Alcohol/drug withdrawal	Other metabolic disturbance, eg hyponatraemia or uraemia

CVA, cerebrovascular accident; SAH, subarachnoid haemorrhage.

History of the presenting problem

This man is clearly not in a position to give an immediate history, but consider the possibilities shown in Table 17.

If the patient remains semi-conscious following termination of his fit, then useful information may be obtained from the following.

- Ambulance crew/notes.

- Medic Alert bracelet or necklace: look carefully at any jewellery.

- Other clues: is he carrying any identification, medication or prescription cards that might suggest he is a known epileptic or diabetic?

- Emergency Department staff: many patients with epilepsy are regular attenders. Does anyone recognise him?

When discussion can take place with the patient or someone who knows him, then if he is a known epileptic it will be important to pursue reasons for the development of status epilepticus. Has he been taking his medication (some epileptics are reluctant to accept their diagnosis)? Has he had an intercurrent illness that has prevented him from taking his medication or which may have altered its absorption (eg gastroenteritis)? Have there been any other changes in his medication that might have altered drug levels?

Is there an underlying cause for the epilepsy that is progressing (eg cerebral space-occupying lesion)? Has he taken large amounts of alcohol or non-prescription drugs that have precipitated the attack?

Examination

The general approach to the examination of the patient in coma is discussed in Section 1.2.31, but particular points to note in this case would include the following.

- Poor general nutrition or hygiene: may indicate alcohol or drug abuse, or (less likely) disseminated malignancy.

- Signs of chronic liver disease due to alcohol abuse, eg spider naevi, jaundice, Dupuytren's contractures and bruising.

- Signs of drug abuse, eg track marks.

- Glasgow Coma Scale score and focal neurological signs: pupillary signs and asymmetry of limb movements may be abnormal following a fit, but persistent asymmetry strongly suggests a focal intracranial lesion.

Investigation

The first investigation of the patient presenting with status epilepticus should be measurement of fingerprick blood glucose to exclude hypoglycaemia. The requirement for further investigation will depend on

the patient's response to immediate treatment to terminate the fit. The known epileptic who responds rapidly and wakes up to give an account that explains events ('I've stopped taking my tablets') does not require extensive investigation. When this is not the case, consider the following.

Routine tests

- Laboratory glucose.

- Electrolytes/renal/liver/bone profile: hyponatraemia, hypocalcaemia and hypomagnesaemia can cause fits, as can hepatic encephalopathy or advanced renal failure.

- FBC.

- Clotting: impairment increases risk of intracerebral haemorrhage.

- Anticonvulsant levels.

- CXR: may show cause of status, eg malignancy that has metastasised to the brain, or complication, eg aspiration pneumonia.

Imaging

CT and/or MRI are warranted in almost all cases of unexplained status epilepticus, but patients should only be moved from the Emergency Department once they have been stabilised.

Other tests

If there is suspicion of an infective cause, then this should be pursued, eg blood cultures, lumbar puncture (if there is no contraindication on CT), thick film for malaria and MRI scanning (Fig. 39) as appropriate.

Arterial blood gases can usefully document the adequacy of oxygenation and ventilation, and may also reveal unexpected metabolic acidosis, which gives a

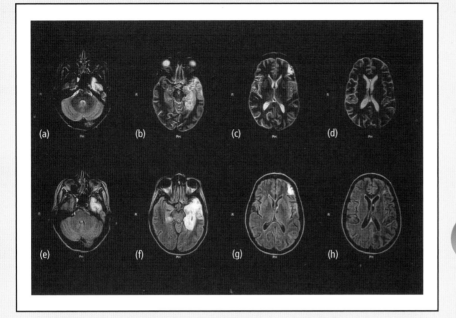

▲**Fig. 39** MRI of herpes simplex encephalitis showing classical cortical distribution mainly in the temporal and parietal lobes: (**a–d**) T2-weighted images; (**e–h**) fluid-attenuated inverse response (FLAIR) images.

Introduction

The working diagnosis must be that this woman has had a stroke, although other conditions must be considered (Table 18). She has some difficulty with speech, described (perhaps loosely) in the scenario as being 'slurred', and so obtaining a history from her may be difficult. First consider whether she has dysphasia.

🔑 **Assess whether patients who might have had a stroke are dysphasic before trying to take a history.**

- Is speech fluent?
- Do they have any receptive dysphasia: can they obey a one-, then two-, then three-step command?
- Do they have any expressive dysphasia, eg nominal dysphasia?

History of the presenting problem

If a history can be obtained from the patient or her husband, ask about the following.

- Onset of symptoms: strokes come on suddenly, so a weakness of gradual onset would suggest a space-occupying lesion.

- Associated symptoms: a sudden severe headache preceding the collapse may suggest an SAH or intracerebral haemorrhage. A history of jaw pain and/or temporal tenderness suggests

clue to poisoning as an explanation for fits, eg ethylene glycol (antifreeze).

Electroencephalography may be required, particularly in patients who remain unconscious. The fits may become progressively more subtle in prolonged epilepsy: non-convulsive status epilepticus.

Further management

Specific treatment, if possible, will be determined by the cause of the fitting. Patients who are recovering from a seizure should be nursed in the recovery position with appropriate management of the airway (nasopharyngeal or oral airway; suction), continued high-flow oxygen and close monitoring (vital signs, neurological observations, ECG and oxygen saturation) until fully recovered. A suitable pressure-relieving mattress, intravenous fluids and urinary catheter will be required if they are slow to regain consciousness.

Referral to a neurologist will be required for optimal long-term

management of epilepsy in appropriate cases.

1.2.30 Stroke

Scenario

A 68-year-old woman is found on the living room floor by her husband. He phones for an ambulance which brings her to the Emergency Department, where she is immediately observed to have right-sided weakness and slurred speech. She has a long history of poorly controlled hypertension. You are asked to assess her.

TABLE 18 DIFFERENTIAL DIAGNOSIS OF STROKE

Common	Must consider
Thrombotic stroke	Subdural haematoma
Embolic stroke	Giant-cell arteritis
Subarachnoid haemorrhage (SAH)	Hypoglycaemia
	Aortic/carotid dissection
	Encephalitis/meningitis
	Cerebral abscess
	Cerebral tumour (primary or secondary)

giant-cell arteritis. Has she been pyrexial? If so, consider unusual cerebral pathology such as brain abscess (commonly spread from infection in the sinuses or middle ear) or meningitis.

Other relevant history

Previous medical history
Have there been any preceding episodes? Ask particularly about amaurosis fugax and transient ischaemic attacks. This woman is hypertensive, but are there any other risk factors for cerebrovascular disease, eg cardiovascular disease, peripheral vascular disease, smoking or diabetes? Is there a history of malignancy that might have led to brain metastasis?

Functional/social history
This woman has only just arrived in the Emergency Department and a range of outcomes, from rapid complete recovery to permanent disability or death, is possible; however, obtaining a social history is important. What was the patient's previous level of functioning? Who else is at home with her and what is the home like (eg does it have stairs)? Although it would clearly be premature to do so at the moment, the earlier a care package can be considered the better, as this is often the primary cause of delays in discharge from hospital and the husband may not be available tomorrow to talk to.

Examination

General features

- Airway, breathing and circulation (ABC).

- Vital signs: has she got a fever? If so, this is most probably due to a

secondary infection as a result of the stroke (eg pneumonia) and much less likely due to the primary cause of the 'stroke' (eg cerebral abscess). Check her pulse: is she in atrial fibrillation? Check her BP: patients are often hypertensive after a stroke, but cerebral autoregulation is also impaired and antihypertensive agents should not be given except in extreme circumstances (see below).

- Cardiovascular: are there any murmurs? Could this be an embolic stroke from endocarditis (look for stigmata)? Are there carotid bruits or other evidence of vascular disease, ie other arterial bruits or absent peripheral pulses? Could there be an aortic dissection (feel both radial pulses and check her BP in both arms if they are not clearly equal)?

- Respiratory: check adequacy of ventilation and for evidence of aspiration.

Neurological system
The important issues to check include the following.

- Glasgow Coma Scale (GCS) score to establish baseline condition.

- Neck stiffness: if present, the diagnosis is likely to be primary SAH.

- Focal signs: to determine the approximate site of the lesion (Table 19).

- Swallowing: dysphagia affects 35% of stroke patients, but is often unrecognised after a mild stroke. It is associated with poor outcome, partly because it predisposes to aspiration and pneumonia, and partly because difficulty with eating leads to starvation.

Can the patient with a stroke eat and drink?

The presence of a gag reflex is a poor guide to safe swallowing and formal assessment by trained staff is essential. Fluids are more difficult to swallow than semi-solids.

Investigation

Imaging
CT scan of the brain should be performed urgently in patients presenting within 3 hours after the onset of symptoms, some of whom may benefit from thrombolysis. Patients presenting after this time also require scanning to distinguish between infarction and haemorrhage, and this can occasionally demonstrate other clinically unsuspected pathologies.

Other routine investigations

- Fingerprick blood glucose.

- FBC: note polycythaemia or thrombocytopenia.

- Clotting screen.

- Inflammatory markers: consider giant-cell arteritis if these are grossly elevated without other explanation.

- Laboratory glucose.

- Electrolytes and renal/liver/bone profiles.

- CXR: aspiration, occasionally another pathology.

- ECG: to exclude dysrhythmias and to look for evidence of recent myocardial infarction.

About 5% of myocardial infarctions in the elderly present with stroke.

TABLE 19 OXFORDSHIRE COMMUNITY STROKE STUDY CLASSIFICATION SYSTEM

Syndrome	Neurological deficit	Cause
Total anterior circulation syndrome (TACS)	New higher cerebral dysfunction (eg dysphasia, dyscalculia and visuospatial disorder) *and* Homonymous visual field defect *and* Ipsilateral motor and/or sensory deficit involving at least two of three areas of the face, arm or leg	Large cortical stroke in middle cerebral, or middle and anterior cerebral artery territories
Partial anterior circulation syndrome (PACS)	Two of the three components of TACS *or* New higher cerebral dysfunction alone *or* Motor/sensory deficit more restricted than those classified as LACS (eg isolated hand involvement)	Cortical stroke in middle or anterior cerebral artery territory
Lacunar syndrome (LACS)	Pure motor stroke *or* Pure sensory stroke *or* Sensorimotor stroke *or* Ataxic hemiparesis *or* Dysarthria and clumsy hand Note that evidence of higher cortical involvement or disturbance of consciousness excludes a lacunar syndrome	Subcortical stroke due to small-vessel disease
Posterior circulation syndrome (POCS)	Ipsilateral cranial nerve palsy with contralateral motor and/or sensory deficit *or* Bilateral motor and/or sensory deficit *or* Disorder of conjugate eye movement *or* Cerebellar dysfunction without ipsilateral pyramidal tract involvement *or* Isolated homonymous visual field defect	Stroke in posterior circulation, brainstem or cortex

Management

🔑 The priorities in management of all patients with acute brain injury are to minimise secondary brain damage and maximise potential recovery.

🔑 **Resuscitation status**

It is vital to assess and clearly record this in the patient's notes: the decision on what the patient's resuscitation status is should be made by a senior member of the medical team after discussion with the patient (where clinical condition allows).

Immediate management

- Secure airway, breathing and oxygenation: nurse the patient in the recovery position if there is impairment of consciousness.

Give high-flow oxygen (hypoxia may be due to aspiration, atelectasis or a reduced central drive to ventilation) aiming to elevate oxygen saturation above 92%. Patients with GCS score <12 may benefit from a nasal or oral airway; those with GCS score <8 need to be considered for elective intubation.

- Obtain intravenous access and give intravenous fluids until the patient's swallow has been assessed as safe; treat hypoglycaemia promptly.

- Consider thrombolysis, but only if there is an agreed hospital protocol and experienced staff (Table 20).

⚠️ Thrombolysis for stroke is an emerging treatment, but should only be given in specialist units.

Continuing management

The outcome is best if the patient can be admitted to a stroke unit for initial acute management as well as rehabilitation.

- General care: nurse on a pressure-relieving mattress; a urinary conveen or catheter may be required; and full-length thromboembolic disease stockings should be applied to prevent deep vein thrombosis, along with early mobilisation if possible.

- Hydration and feeding: dysphagic patients should be fed through a nasogastric tube or percutaneous endoscopic feeding tube until it is safe to resume oral food and fluids.

- Glycaemic control: hyperglycaemia should be prevented, if necessary using a sliding scale of intravenous insulin. Good glycaemic control

---

TABLE 20 SUGGESTED GUIDELINES FOR THE USE OF INTRAVENOUS RECOMBINANT TISSUE PLASMINOGEN ACTIVATOR IN ISCHAEMIC STROKE

Guideline	Comment
Indication	Consider in all patients with proven ischaemic stroke presenting within 3 hours of onset
Clinical exclusion criteria	Use of oral anticoagulants and/or INR >1.7 Use of heparin in the preceding 48 hours or prolonged partial thromboplastin time Platelet count <100 × 10^9/L Stroke or serious head injury in the previous 3 months Major surgery within the previous 14 days Pretreatment systolic BP >185 mmHg or diastolic BP >110 mmHg Rapidly improving neurological condition Mild isolated neurological deficits Previous intracranial haemorrhage Blood glucose >22 mmol/L or <2.8 mmol/L Seizure at stroke onset Gastrointestinal or urinary bleeding within the previous 21 days Recent myocardial infarction
Clinical caution	Severe stroke: National Institutes of Health stroke scale score >22
Radiological contraindication	CT suggests early changes of major infarction, eg sulcal effacement, mass effect or oedema
Clinical requirement	Thrombolytic therapy should only be administered by physicians with expertise in stroke medicine who have access to a suitable stroke service with facilities for identifying and managing haemorrhagic complications. It is recommended that treatment and its adverse effects are discussed with the patient and/or the family before treatment
Regimen	Recombinant tissue plasminogen activator 0.9 mg/kg iv, up to a maximum of 90 mg; the first 10% as a bolus, the rest as an infusion over 60 minutes

---

improves the outcome from acute stroke.

- Aspirin: should be given (oral, nasogastric tube and rectal preparations are available) when haemorrhagic stroke has been excluded.

BP commonly increases following acute stroke and settles over the next 24–48 hours. Immediate attempts to lower the pressure are much more likely to do harm than good: cerebral autoregulation is disturbed and rapid reduction of BP may reduce cerebral perfusion below a critical threshold. Most would recommend gentle pressure reduction only if the systolic is consistently above 220 mmHg or the diastolic above 130 mmHg, with modified-release nifedipine 10 mg po stat being a suitable initial treatment. In the rare case of stroke associated with malignant hypertension, the BP needs to be lowered slowly: use an intravenous agent such as labetalol and aim to reduce BP by 25% over the next 24 hours.

The patient should be referred to ancillary services sooner rather than later: speech therapy, physiotherapy, occupational therapy and the social work department. Secondary prevention (apart from BP control) should be started soon after admission, including the need to stop smoking.

Further comments

Depending on the outcome from the stroke, further investigation may be appropriate for selected cases. In young stroke patients make sure that you obtain an accurate drug/social history (amphetamine and cocaine), consider detailed thrombophilia testing (eg lupus anticoagulant) and pursue possible cardiac sources of emboli (echocardiography, transthoracic and transoesphageal). Carotid Doppler studies should be performed if the patient would be a suitable candidate for surgery.

1.2.31 Coma

Scenario

A man of about 40 years who lives alone has not been seen for 2 days. His neighbours go to his house to investigate, find him collapsed and call an emergency ambulance. The paramedics give oxygen, obtain venous access and bring him to the Emergency Department where you are asked to assess him. He is unconscious. The neighbours have not accompanied him to hospital.

Immediate management

In the first 5 minutes of dealing with an unconscious patient the priorities are as follows

- Assess and manage airway, breathing, circulation (ABC): if the main problem is with A, B or C, then proceed as described in Sections 1.2.1 and 1.2.2.

- Give high-flow oxygen; apply pulse oximeter to monitor oxygen saturation.

- Obtain intravenous access (if not already established).

- Consider hypoglycaemia: check fingerprick blood glucose; if <2.5 mmol/L give 50 mL of 50% dextrose intravenously (see Section 1.2.21).

- Consider opioid toxicity: check pupils and respiratory rate. If the pupils are small and the respiratory rate is low, give naloxone 400 μg iv stat, repeated up to a total of 1.2 mg if there is a response.

- Check temperature: is the patient hypothermic? Always use a low-reading thermometer and measure the rectal temperature (axillary, skin, tympanic and oral temperatures are often inaccurate in this setting). If the patient is hypothermic, start rewarming.

- Check score on Glasgow Coma Scale (GCS) (Fig. 40) and look for localising neurological signs: facial asymmetry; movement of right arm and leg compared with left arm and leg; size and reaction of pupils; and abnormal eye position, gaze or eye movements.

- Consider Wernicke's encephalopathy, especially if there are signs of alcohol abuse, and if this is a possibility give intravenous thiamine (see Section 1.2.18).

> **Check fingerprick blood glucose immediately in any patient in coma.**

> **The half-lives of most opioids are longer than that of naloxone: patients in coma from opioid overdose often require repeated doses of naloxone or an infusion.**

History of the presenting problem

The unconscious patient will clearly not be able to give a history, but consider the diagnoses listed in Table 21 as you gather information from any source that you can.

Details of the precise circumstances at the scene where the patient was found are required, either from the ambulance crew (or their written notes) or from the neighbours if they subsequently come to the hospital. Also, any information about the patient's general health/past medical history is very important. Is he known to have diabetes or epilepsy, or any other major medical problem? Is he known to take any regular medications? Where was he found? If at the foot of the stairs, it would suggest a fall. Were there any drug bottles or syringes nearby? What was the state of the surroundings? Was the house well kept? Was there any suggestion of carbon monoxide poisoning? Had a suicide note been left?

Examination

Look for the following in particular after initiating the immediate management described above.

Glasgow Coma Scale

Best eye opening response	Score
Spontaneously	4
To speech	3
To pain	2
None	1

Best verbal response	
Orientated	5
Confused conversation	4
Words	3
Sounds	2
None	1

Best motor response	
Obeys commands	6
Localisation to painful stimuli	5
Withdraws to pain	4
Flexor (decorticate) response to pain	3
Extensor (decerebrate) response to pain	2
No response	1

Notes
- Maximum score is 15, minimum is 3; coma is defined as 8 or less; significant deterioration is defined as a decrease in GCS score of 2 or more. Record components separately, e.g. patient with GCS 8 may be E2, V2, M4.
- Motor response should be scored as the best response of any limb.
- Painful stimuli: do not use methods that might lead to bleeding or bruising. The best techniques are to apply pressure to a nail-bed by squeezing a pencil or biro hard against it, and by rubbing the sternum hard with your knuckles.

▲**Fig. 40** Glasgow Coma Scale.

TABLE 21 DIFFERENTIAL DIAGNOSIS OF COMA

Frequency[1]	Condition
Common	Hypoglycaemia
	Opioid toxicity
	Head injury
	Post ictal
	Subarachnoid haemorrhage (SAH)
	Stroke
	Alcohol
Less common/rare	Other poisoning: benzodiazepine, tricyclic antidepressant or carbon monoxide
	Other intracranial haemorrhage: extradural or subdural
	Hypothermia
	Metabolic: hyponatraemia, hepatic encephalopathy or advanced renal failure
	Infective: encephalitis, meningitis or malaria
	Non-convulsive status

1. Frequency is as in UK practice; head injury is usually obvious, but not always.

Head-to-toe screen

- General condition: poor nutrition or hygiene may indicate alcohol or drug abuse in this context.

- Signs of chronic liver disease: likely to be due to alcohol abuse.

- Signs of drug abuse, eg track marks.

- Signs of trauma: either as a primary cause of the collapse (feel the back of the head and neck for bruising/induration) or as a consequence of it (check for features of pressure necrosis and compartment syndromes).

- Respiratory pattern: Cheyne–Stokes respiration is associated with bilateral cortical damage; hyperventilation may occur secondary to metabolic acidosis, pulmonary pathology or, rarely, brainstem pathology; and bizarre respiratory patterns may be associated with brainstem pathology.

Neurological

- Pupillary size and reaction: bilateral fixed and dilated pupils suggest severe damage and are a very poor prognostic sign (but ensure the patient is not wearing cosmetic contact lenses). A unilateral, fixed and dilated pupil indicates a third nerve lesion, commonly due to uncal herniation from a supratentorial mass lesion or a posterior communicating artery aneurysm. Unilateral Horner's syndrome suggests damage to the hypothalamus or a lateral medullary syndrome. Bilateral small pupils suggest opioid overdose or more rarely pontine damage.

- Eye movements: abnormal conjugate deviation suggests intracerebral damage. Disconjugate deviation implies damage to cranial nerves III, IV or VI.

- Asymmetry of peripheral tone or reflexes suggests focal neurological damage.

Investigation

Glucose and imaging

The first investigation in the unconscious patient should always be a fingerprick blood glucose. If the patient's GCS score is falling, indicating deterioration, or there are focal neurological signs, then the next priority is to organise an urgent CT scan of the brain, which may reveal something that requires immediate neurosurgical attention.

⚠ Do not send patients in coma for a CT scan without ensuring that ABC are secure and that a suitably experienced member of staff accompanies them.

Other routine tests

FBC, clotting, electrolytes, laboratory glucose and a renal/liver/bone profile may give an indication of some of the conditions listed in Table 21. Perform a CXR to rule out aspiration. About 80% of patients who have had an SAH have ECG changes, which in around 10% suggests an acute myocardial infarction.

Other tests in selected cases

Blood cultures will be appropriate is there is clinical suspicion of sepsis, and thick films for malaria are necessary in cases with the possibility of exposure. Lumbar puncture may be required, after CT, in selected patients. Aside from confirming oxygenation and ventilation, arterial blood gases may show metabolic acidosis, a critical clue to the fact that a patient's coma is due to poisoning (see Section 1.2.36).

Management

Specific management will clearly depend on the cause of coma, and you should have a low threshold for treating unlikely but plausible treatable causes, eg aciclovir if herpes simplex encephalitis is possible.

Patients who remain in coma after initial resuscitation measures have been undertaken will require transfer to an intensive care unit. Those who recover to a GCS score of ≥8 may be managed in a suitable high-dependency area; there they should be nursed in the recovery position with appropriate management of the airway (nasopharyngeal or oral airway, suction) and continued high-flow oxygen until fully recovered, along with ECG and oxygen saturation monitoring and regular neurological and systemic observations. A suitable pressure-relieving mattress, intravenous fluids and a urinary convene/catheter will be required.

1.2.32 Fever in a returning traveller

Scenario

A 25-year-old man is brought to the Emergency Department by his friends. He has recently returned from a back-packing trip around Thailand and has not been well since his return. He is drowsy and has a temperature of 39°C. You are asked to review him immediately on his arrival.

Introduction

Malaria

- Consider malaria in *any* patient presenting to hospital with coma and/or fever and a relevant travel history.
- There are no diagnostic findings on examination.
- Missing the diagnosis can be fatal.

Malaria must be the working diagnosis in this man. Falciparum malaria is usually the cause of severe, complicated malaria. Cerebral malaria, a complication of *Plasmodium falciparum* infection, may present with coma. There will probably be an antecedent history of a short febrile illness with rigors and headache. Patients infected with *Plasmodium vivax*, *Plasmodium ovale* or *Plasmodium malariae* tend to have milder symptoms. The incubation period is at least 7 days, but remember that vivax and ovale malaria can cause symptoms for the first time more than 12 months after infection.

Other diagnoses

The diagnosis is malaria! However, be wary: Gram-negative sepsis commonly coexists with malaria and typhoid in particular must be considered. Meningitis may be the only manifestation of typhoid, when it may resemble any other pyogenic meningitis. Consider a broad differential including fungal, viral and other protozoal infections. Also consider encephalitis and cerebral abcess, and drug ingestion may be complicating the picture.

History of the presenting problem

This man may be too unwell to give a lucid account but if he is able to then, aside from routine enquiry about how the illness began, how it progressed, localising symptoms and past medical history, the most important issues in this case are clearly to get a full travel and social history to establish which pathogens the patient may have been exposed to, and whether precautions to prevent infection have been taken. Ask about:

- countries visited and when;
- areas visited (rural or urban, rainforest or savannah);
- accommodation used;
- activities whilst there, eg freshwater exposure or trekking;
- exposure to animals;
- sexual history;
- vaccinations received prior to travel;
- antimalarial chemoprophylaxis and compliance.

⚠️ Malaria can cause misleading localising features such as abdominal pain, diarrhoea, breathlessness or jaundice.

⚠️ The fact that a patient has taken malaria prophylaxis does not rule out malaria: it is 70–90% effective (if taken).

Examination

The general approaches to investigation of the patient who is very ill or in coma are discussed in Sections 1.2.2 and 1.2.31. Malaria produces no diagnostic physical signs. Anaemia and slight jaundice are common, with moderate tender hepatosplenomegaly. There is no rash or lymphadenopathy.

Investigation

An immediate thick and thin malaria film is required (Fig. 41). Remember that a single negative film does not exclude malaria: it is very unlikely if three films are negative, although it cannot be completely excluded until another diagnosis is made or the illness resolves.

The approach to investigation of the patient who is very ill and/or has suspected sepsis is described in Sections 1.2.2 and 1.2.27. Note that anaemia, leucopenia, thrombocytopenia, abnormal clotting, renal failure and deranged liver function may all be seen with malaria.

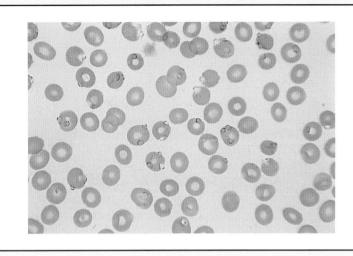

▲ **Fig. 41** Malaria film showing falciparum malaria.

Management

> If you are not familiar with the management of malaria, seek expert advice sooner rather than later, particularly if the patient has been to northern Thailand, Laos or Burma as there is a high incidence of quinine resistance in these areas and combination therapy may be required.

The general approaches to management of the patient who is very ill or in coma are discussed in Sections 1.2.2 and 1.2.31. With regard to the patient with malaria, note the following.

- Hypoglycaemia is common in severe malaria: monitor blood glucose hourly and give intravenous dextrose if necessary.

- Remember that there is a clear association between bacterial infection and malaria: in addition to treatment for malaria, treat the patient empirically with broad-spectrum antibiotics after taking blood cultures if they are seriously ill.

Drug treatment of malaria

Falciparum malaria If the patient can swallow, first-line treatment is now Riamet (each tablet contains artemether 20 mg with lumefantrine 120 mg), four tablets twice daily for 3 days. The 'standard' alternative, which remains the treatment of choice in many countries, is quinine 600 mg (of salt) three times daily for 7 days, followed by a single dose of three tablets of Fansidar (sulfadoxine/pyramethamine) or doxycycline 100 mg daily for 7 days.

If the patient cannot swallow, give intravenous quinine (loading dose 20 mg/kg of dihydrochloride salt, maximum 1400 mg, over 4 hours; then 10 mg/kg over 4 hours twice daily), intravenous artesunate or intramuscular artemether. Omit the loading dose of quinine if the patient has received mefloquine witin the last week or quinine has been given in the last 24 hours.

While the quinine is being administered make sure that the patient is on a cardiac monitor and the fingerprick blood glucose is measured hourly.

Vivax, ovale and malariae malaria
Give oral chloroquine 600 mg immediately, followed after 6 hours by 300 mg and then two further doses of 300 mg at 24- and 48-hour intervals. In vivax and ovale infections, chloroquine should then be followed by a 2-week course of primaquine 15 mg daily to eliminate parasites from the liver.

> ⚠ Remember to screen patients for glucose-6-phosphate dehydrogenase deficiency before giving primaquine otherwise severe haemolysis may ensue.

Further comment

See *Infectious Diseases*, Sections 1.3.16 and 2.13.1 for more detailed discussion of this presentation and the management of malaria.

1.2.33 Anaphylaxis

Scenario

A 40-year-old woman has been admitted to the ward for treatment of a community-acquired pneumonia. Shortly after taking the first dose of amoxicillin she complains of difficulty breathing and of swollen lips and tongue. The nurses have put out a 'cardiac arrest' call. You are the leader of the cardiac arrest team and are expected to manage the patient.

Introduction

> **Anaphylaxis**
>
> Anaphylaxis is a severe allergic reaction to an allergen that the patient has previously been exposed to. It is mediated by antigen-specific cross-linking of IgE molecules on the surface of tissue mast cells and peripheral blood basophils.

Anaphylactoid reactions

Anaphylactoid reactions are an immediate systemic reaction that mimic anaphylaxis but which are not mediated by IgE and may occur on first exposure to the allergen.

For life-threatening anaphylaxis, consider injection of slow intravenous epinephrine (adrenaline) 1 in 10,000 solution (note the 10-fold dilution compared with the intramuscular injection): give 5 mL (0.5 mg) at a rate of 1 mL/min until a response has been obtained.

Immediate management

This woman is clearly having an anaphylactic reaction.

- Assess airway, breathing and circulation (ABC).

- Give high-flow oxygen via a reservoir bag and apply a pulse oximeter to monitor oxygen saturation.

- Give epinephrine (adrenaline) if there is stridor, wheeze, respiratory distress or clinical signs of shock: the initial dose is 0.5 mL of 1 in 1,000 solution intramuscularly, repeated in 5 minutes if there is no improvement.

- Obtain intravenous access.

- Give chlorpheniramine 10–20 mg im or iv.

- Give hydrocortisone 100–500 mg iv.

- Give salbutamol 5–10 mg by nebuliser if bronchospasm is present.

- Give 0.9% saline 1 L stat if the patient is hypotensive.

If confronted by a patient *in extremis*, call for help immediately. Do not wait until the heart has stopped before putting out a cardiac arrest call.

History of the presenting problem

In this case the history of exposure to a precipitant is clear-cut and it is extremely unlikely that the diagnosis is anything other than an anaphylactic reaction to amoxicillin, although the patient may also have received other drugs during admission. However, in many instances of anaphylaxis it is not clear what the precipitant is, in which case it is important to discuss the following issues if and when the patient is able to give a history.

- Is there a previous history of allergy or anaphylaxis?

- Exactly what allergen has precipitated the attack? Many different substances can precipitate anaphylaxis so it is necessary to talk through events in the hour or so preceding the attack in minute detail. Ask the following questions: 'What have you eaten and drunk? Anything else? No nuts [a common precipitant]? Have you been bitten or stung by anything? Have you been exposed to rubber or latex? What medications are you taking [salicylates and angiotensin-converting enzyme inhibitors are the most likely culprits]? Have there been any recent changes to these? Have you taken any non-prescription drugs from any source?'

- Is there a family history of allergy/anaphylaxis (consider C1 inhibitor deficiency)?

Examination, investigation and further management

The approach to the examination, investigation and management of the patient who is extremely ill is discussed in Sections 1.2.1 and 1.2.2, but note the following with regard to the patient with anaphylaxis.

- Serum mast cell tryptase: elevated following anaphylaxis and useful for confirming the diagnosis when there is clinical doubt.

Patients should always be admitted for observation, even if they show an initial good response to treatment. Problems can recur several hours later, especially following ingestion of an allergen or an insect bite.

Further comments

Patients with anaphylaxis should be referred for specialist advice. This may help to identify the allergen, and they may need instruction on the use of self-administered epinephrine (EpiPen).

All patients with a history of anaphylaxis should be encouraged to wear a Medic-Alert necklace or bracelet.

See *Acute Medicine*, Section 1.2.33, and *Rheumatology and Clinical Immunology*, Section 1.4.2 for further discussion.

1.2.34 A painful joint

Scenario

A 45-year-old woman presents to the Emergency Department with a painful hot knee. She has previously been diagnosed by her GP as having 'probable rheumatoid arthritis', but this has not been a problem for many years. She is afebrile, her pulse is 80 bpm and her BP is 150/75 mmHg. You are asked to see and assess her knee.

TABLE 22 DIFFERENTIAL DIAGNOSIS OF AN ACUTE HOT JOINT

Frequency	Type of condition	Example
Common	Crystal arthritis	Gout Pseudogout
	Infectious	Non-gonococcal septic arthritis caused by pyogenic bacteria: *Staphylococcus aureus* (70%), other Gram-positive cocci (20%), Gram-negative bacilli (10%)
	Post-infectious	Reactive arthritis
Less common	Bleeding	Haemarthrosis
	Inflammatory	Other spondyloarthritides (not reactive arthritis)
	Infectious	Gonococcal arthritis (rare in the UK, more common in the USA and Australasia) Lyme disease Tuberculosis
Rare	Inflammatory	Monoarticular presentation of rheumatoid arthritis (RA) Palindromic RA
	Other	Osteonecrosis (especially involving the hip)

Introduction

Joint pain is a common symptom that may be a manifestation of a variety of rheumatic disorders, including those caused by inflammation, cartilage degeneration, crystal deposition, infection and trauma. It may be a localised manifestation of a systemic disorder. Consider the diagnoses given in Table 22 as you pursue the history and examination.

History of the presenting problem

The following features in the history would aid you in making a diagnosis in someone presenting with a single painful joint.

- Time course of onset: an abrupt onset is when joint symptoms develop over minutes to hours and may be caused by trauma, crystal synovitis or infection. An insidious onset, when joint symptoms develop over weeks to months, is typical of most forms of arthritis, including RA and osteoarthritis.

- Are other joints involved? Monoarthritis (the involvement of one joint) would be typical of the conditions listed in Table 22; oligoarthritis (the involvement of two to four joints) or polyarthritis (the involvement of five or more joints) would suggest RA, psoriatic arthropathy or other autoimmune rheumatic diseases.

- Symmetry of joint involvement: symmetrical arthritis, characterised by involvement of the same joints on each side of the body, is typical of RA, systemic lupus erythematosus and other autoimmune rheumatic diseases. Psoriatic arthritis, reactive arthritis (Reiter's syndrome) and Lyme arthritis typically present asymmetrically.

- Nature of the pain: with inflammatory joint disease the pain is present both at rest and with motion, being worse at the beginning of usage and improving as the patient gets 'warmed up'; with non-inflammatory (ie degenerative, traumatic or mechanical) joint disease the pain occurs mainly or only during motion and improves quickly with rest. Patients with advanced degenerative disease of the hips, spine or knees may also have pain at rest and at night.

- Stiffness: a perceived sensation of tightness when attempting to move joints after a period of inactivity, which typically subsides over time. Its duration may serve to distinguish inflammatory from non-inflammatory forms of joint disease. With inflammatory arthritis it is present on waking and typically lasts 30–60 minutes or longer. With non-inflammatory arthritis stiffness is experienced briefly (eg 15 minutes) on waking in the morning or following periods of inactivity.

- Swelling: with inflammatory arthritis, joint swelling is related to synovial hypertrophy, synovial effusion and/or inflammation of periarticular structures. The degree of swelling often varies over time. With non-inflammatory arthritis the formation of osteophytes leads to bony swelling.

It is also important to ask about the functional consequences of loss of motion, which may arise due to structural damage, inflammation or contracture of surrounding soft tissues: is the patient limited in any activities of daily living?

Other relevant history

A full general history is required but, noting the conditions listed in Table 22, points of particular interest would include the following.

- History of trauma to the joint.

- Systemic features such as fever, ulcers (orogenital), rashes and eye symptoms.

- Past history of joint problems: this patient is said to have probably had RA. What is the evidence for this?

- Drug history: anticoagulants predispose to intra-articular bleeds and corticosteroid use can result in avascular necrosis.

In appropriate cases a detailed sexual and drug abuse history will be necessary.

Examination

As always begin with an overall assessment of the patient's condition: those with a septic arthritis are usually very ill. On general physical examination take note of the following.

- Temperature.

- Rash: reactive arthritis commonly occurs with viral illnesses.

- Eyes: are there any signs of conjunctivitis or uveitis?

- Presence of tophi.

- Consider examination of the external genitalia for ulceration/discharge.

With regard to the knee:

- inspect and palpate for swelling, erythema, synovial effusion and warmth, comparing the affected joint with the contralateral one;

- check motion – synovitis with or without a synovial effusion may result in a decrease in the range, including a loss of full extension (flexion deformity) and/or a reduction in flexion;

- palpate for crepitus with passive movement.

Investigation

> The first priority in dealing with an acute hot joint is to rule out septic arthritis.

Joint aspiration

The single most useful and important test is joint aspiration: send synovial fluid for urgent microscopy (white blood cell count, Gram stain and polarising microscopy for crystals of gout or pseudogout) and culture (Table 23). The finding of non-inflammatory joint fluid in an acutely inflamed joint should prompt consideration of another pathology (eg stress fracture, osteomyelitis or avascular necrosis), acute inflammation of periarticular structures (eg gouty inflammation of tendon sheaths or bursae, septic bursitis) or subcutaneous inflammation (eg cellulites).

> Aside from being crucial to obtaining a diagnosis, aspiration of a hot joint often provides considerable pain relief.

Other tests

Blood cultures should be taken in all cases and a clotting screen performed if there is haemarthrosis. Other tests rarely provide very useful information in patients with a single hot joint: the white cell count may be raised in infection; elevation of inflammatory markers (erythrocyte sedimentation rate and C-reactive protein) is non-specific; the level of serum uric acid is uninformative about whether gout is the problem; testing for autoantibodies is rarely revealing; and joint radiographs are usually unhelpful, although chondrocalcinosis may be seen in pseudogout.

Management

Specific treatment will depend on the diagnosis, but note the following.

Analgesia

NSAIDs should initially be given at their maximum recommended dosage until symptoms improve, after which they should be tapered gradually over several days. Indometacin is very effective, but adverse effects in some patients limit its utility; other NSAIDs with short half-lives (eg ibuprofen and diclofenac) can also be used.

Colchicine has a narrow therapeutic window that limits its effectiveness, and its use in treating acute gouty arthritis (as opposed to being used in low doses to prevent attacks) has been largely supplanted by other therapies.

Corticosteroids are an effective alternative to NSAIDs and colchicine for patients in whom these drugs may be contraindicated or hazardous (eg patients of advanced age or with renal insufficiency, congestive heart failure or an inability to take oral medications). Regimens include:

TABLE 23 FINDINGS ON ASPIRATION OF SYNOVIAL FLUID

Condition	Macroscopic appearance	White cell count ($\times 10^9$/L)	Polymorphonuclear neutrophils
Normal	Clear	0–0.2	<10%
Non-inflammatory	Clear	0.2–2.0	<20%
Inflammatory	Slightly turbid	2.0–50	20–70%
Pyo-arthrosis	Turbid	>50	>70%

- intramuscular injection of a long-acting crystalline preparation (eg triamcinolone 60–80 mg), with an option to repeat once after 24–48 hours;

- prednisolone 20–30 mg/day with progressive tapering over 7–10 days;

- intra-articular corticosteroid therapy.

Opiates are very likely to be needed for patients with septic arthritis, and appropriate joint support and positioning should not be neglected.

Antibiotics

If there is purulent synovial fluid or organisms on the patient's Gram stain, then request an orthopaedic opinion (joint wash-out may be appropriate) and give high-dose flucloxacillin plus a third-generation cephalosporin, which can be withdrawn if cultures are negative at 24 hours. The minimum period of antibiotic treatment for septic arthritis is 6 weeks (usually with 2 weeks intravenously initially).

See *Rheumatology and Clinical Immunology*, Section 1.4.4 for further discussion.

1.2.35 Back pain

Scenario

A 35-year-old man presents with acute low back pain. This came on when he lifted up his 3-year-old son and has now been present for 2 days. On getting dressed today he experienced the sudden onset of severe pain and has since been unable to move. He called an ambulance and has been brought to the Medical Admissions Unit where you have been asked to assess and hopefully to discharge him.

Introduction

Back pain is exceedingly common and not usually caused by sinister disease, but you must be aware of 'red flags' and pursue appropriate investigations if these are present. If they are not, then you should not investigate unnecessarily but reassure the patient and provide effective analgesia.

History of the presenting problem

Simple mechanical back pain

This typically affects the lower back and can be referred to the buttocks and thighs; it varies with posture or activity and alters over time in response to altered activities or treatment. The referred pain is usually dull and poorly localised; it can affect both legs.

Nerve root or radicular pain

This is usually the patient's main complaint when present. It is sharp and well localised, following a dermatome quite closely, and is often associated with sensations of numbness or tingling. Nerve root pain at the common L5 and S1 levels usually extends to the foot or toes.

'Sciatica' is a lay term for pain and sensations of tingling that travel into the buttocks, back of the thigh and into the calf and heel. These symptoms are caused by irritation of the sciatic nerve. Non-specific pain from the lumbar area can also be referred in the distribution of the sciatic nerve.

Red flags

It is essential to check for 'red flags', which increase the chance of the diagnosis being something other than simple mechanical low back pain.

'Red flags' in the patient with back pain

- Age under 20 or over 55 years.
- History of malignancy, steroids, intravenous drug use, HIV or other significant past history.
- Systemic symptoms such as fever or weight loss.
- Progressive neurological deficit, eg saddle anaesthesia, sphincteric disturbance, other motor or sensory deficits.
- Structural deformity.
- Persistent night pain.
- Thoracic pain.

Examination

A screening general examination will be required, but attention will properly focus on examination of the back and for neurological signs in the legs. Beware the patient with back pain who looks ill with evidence of circulatory compromise: there may be a leaking abdominal aortic aneurysm.

Remember that back pain may be caused by a leaking abdominal aortic aneurysm.

The back

Look for deformity or local tenderness of the back, and perform the passive straight leg raise test (PSLT) for diagnosing nerve root pain due to herniated discs, for which it has high sensitivity (about 90%) but low specificity (about 20%). With the person lying flat on the back with both legs straight, raise one leg until limited by pain and/or tight hamstrings. Slightly lower the leg to provide relief. In this position, increase tension on the sciatic nerve by dorsiflexion of the foot (or flexion of the

TABLE 24 SENSORY AND MOTOR DEFICITS OF ROOT LESIONS IN THE LEG

Lesion	Sensory deficit	Motor deficit	Tendon jerks
L2	Often none (across upper thigh)	Hip flexion	No defect
L3	Often none (across lower thigh)	Knee extension	Knee jerk reduced/absent
L4	Medial leg	Foot inversion	Knee jerk reduced/absent
L5	Dorsum of foot	Toe dorsiflexion	No defect
S1	Behind lateral malleolus	Foot plantarflexion and eversion	Ankle jerk reduced/absent

neck/compression of the nerve in the popliteal fossa). This will aggravate or elicit pain radiating down the raised leg if there is nerve root irritation. The pain should be relieved by flexion of the knee. The PSLT can also be performed in the sitting position. A discrepancy with the supine PSLT suggests that the symptoms could be factitious.

Neurological examination
Look for focal signs as described in *Clinical Skills for PACES* and shown in Table 24.

Cauda equina syndrome
Saddle anaesthesia, bladder disturbance, faecal incontinence and bilateral numbness or weakness in lower limbs.

Investigation

Only consider diagnostic imaging and other investigations if red flags are present or there is significant fracture risk (owing to trauma, steroids or osteoporosis).

Imaging
Plain radiological films are unhelpful in the acute setting in the absence of red flags or significant fracture risk; MRI is the best procedure for

diagnosing nerve root compression, discitis and neoplasms (Fig. 42).

Other investigations
Patients with simple mechanical back pain should not be investigated. If red flags are present, then investigation should be determined by clinical suspicion.

- Infection: blood cultures, FBC and inflammatory markers; also diagnostic biopsy.

- Malignancy: FBC, inflammatory markers, liver/bone profile, prostate-specific antigen and serum immunoglobulins/serum protein electrophoresis/urinary Bence Jones proteins; CXR and bone scan; and diagnostic biopsy.

- Inflammatory: FBC, inflammatory markers, autoimmune rheumatic serology and human leucocyte antigen (HLA)-B27.

Management

Anyone with symptoms suggestive of cauda equina syndrome needs immediate neurosurgical referral: this is a surgical emergency.

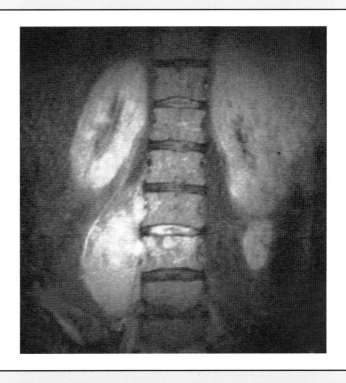

▲**Fig. 42** MRI scan of a patient presenting with a short history of back pain and perianal anaesthesia. The body of L3 and the right psoas muscle are infiltrated. Biopsy revealed high-grade non-Hodgkin's lymphoma.

For those who do not have simple mechanical back pain, specific management will depend on the cause.

Patients with simple mechanical back pain should be given adequate analgesia. Follow the analgesic ladder from simple non-opioids (eg paracetamol) to opioids (eg co-codamol, then morphine), give a co-analgesic (eg NSAID), and use muscle relaxants (eg diazepam 2 mg three times daily) in the early stages. The patient should be discharged home as soon as pain has been reduced to tolerable levels, with instructions to stay active and return to work/usual activities as soon as possible. The prognosis for simple mechanical back pain is good: 90% recover at 6 weeks, although recurrence is common. The prognosis for those with nerve root pain ('sciatica') is less good, with only 50% recovering at 6 weeks.

See *Rheumatology and Clinical Immunology*, Sections 1.1.12 and 1.1.13 for further discussion.

1.2.36 Self-harm

Scenario

A 25-year-old woman is brought to the Emergency Department following an overdose of 30 500-mg paracetamol tablets 9 hours prior to her arrival in hospital. She refuses to say anything other than that she wants to be left alone to die. She has refused all medical intervention. You are asked to see her.

Introduction

Can you treat the patient?
It is common for patients who have intentionally harmed themselves to refuse to stay in hospital or accept treatment. The capacity to consent to medical treatment or make a valid refusal is a legal concept not a medical one, and therefore it is independent of the diagnosis. If this woman is assumed to have full capacity to refuse medical treatment, she may well develop liver failure and possibly die. If patients have such a capacity, it is of no consequence whether you agree with their decision, and whatever their reasons you must respect their decision unless they are detained under the Mental Health Act.

It is reasonable to call on psychiatric services to make an assessment of a patient's capacity, but there is often insufficient time to do this and so you must be able to make this assessment as well. Case law has widely recognised that factors such as drugs, fatigue, panic, pain, shock and confusion will erode a patient's capacity, in which case you will be able to proceed with urgent treatment in good faith, provided you are acting in the patient's best interests and in line with the view of a responsible body of medical opinion. See also Section 1.2.37.

Treating a patient who does not want to be treated

If you believe that a patient who has taken an overdose has a mental illness and assess that his or her capacity is in doubt, your duty of care allows you to undertake treatment despite the patient's opposition and ultimately potentially save the patient's life.

History of the presenting problem
Getting a reliable history from a patient who has taken an overdose can be difficult if not impossible, but to be able to judge the likely medical consequences of an overdose it is clearly necessary to try to establish what has been taken and when. Always presume that other tablets or alcohol have been taken.

Other relevant history
Details of previous medical, psychiatric and social history are required, the main aim of psychiatric assessment being to establish the risk of suicide.

Psychiatric and social background
Is there a past history of deliberate self-harm? Is the patient known to suffer from affective disorder, schizophrenia, alcoholism or drug dependence? Is she socially isolated or recently separated? Have there been any other recent adverse life events? Is there a history of aggressive or impulsive behaviour?

Assessing the risk of suicide
Did she take the overdose on impulse or had she planned it for some time? Features that would suggest planning and a high suicide risk include hoarding of pills, taking precautions to make sure that she was alone and undisturbed when she took the pills, leaving a suicide note, giving away treasured possessions before the event, arranging for children to be sent away and the use of more than one means to try to kill herself.

High-risk clinical factors for suicide

- Severe insomnia.
- Self-neglect.
- Memory impairment.
- Agitation.
- Panic attacks.
- Pessimism, anhedonia, despair and morbid guilt.

> - Patients are not experts in pharmacology: do not assume that a small overdose of a relatively safe drug implies lack of lethal intent.
> - The degree of suicidal intent can fluctuate.
> - Gravely suicidal patients can deliberately conceal their intentions: patients may appear misleadingly calm after they have made a firm but undisclosed plan to kill themselves.

Examination

The immediate priority in any patient presenting with deliberate self-harm is physical examination, beginning with airway, breathing and circulation (ABC) and Glasgow Coma Scale (GCS) score. The approach to the patient who is in circulatory collapse or unconscious is described in Sections 1.2.2 and 1.2.31. When it is possible to examine the mental state the most important aspects include the following.

- Does she exhibit self-neglect, anhedonia, pessimism, guilt, remorse and self-recrimination?

- Does she convey a feeling of helplessness and despair?

- Are there depressive or nihilistic delusions?

- Has she experienced command hallucinations?

- Does she wish that she had not surivived the overdose?

Investigation

Check levels of paracetamol and salicylate in addition to a routine screen of FBC, clotting, electrolytes and renal/liver/bone profile, with other tests if clinically indicated. Urine and serum samples may need to be saved for later toxicological analysis. Check arterial blood gases if the patient is very unwell, has a

GCS score <10 or if ventilation is clinically inadequate.

Management

If the patient is in circulatory shock, then resuscitate as described in Section 1.2.1, and if they have impairment of consciousness then as described in Section 1.2.31. For details of specific management of paracetamol toxicity see Section 2.1.2.

Further comments

Risk of suicide

Patients who present with self-harm are 100 times more at risk of suicide compared with the general population. The medical seriousness of an episode is not necessarily indicative of the suicide risk (although violent methods such as attempted shooting are obviously high risk). Self-harm is the most powerful single predictor for completed suicide.

1.2.37 Violence and aggression

> ### Scenario
>
> Police have brought a 32-year-old man to the Emergency Department because they think him disturbed and a risk to others. He is now aggressive and threatening violence towards hospital staff. You are called to assess him.

Introduction

Common law

> 🔑 Any patient lacking the capacity to consent can be treated under common law.

Nothing can be done for patients without their consent unless you, as a registered medical practitioner, have assessed and documented them as not having the capacity to consent to treatment. The capacity to consent to or refuse medical treatment requires patients to understand what is happening, why it is happening and what may happen if they refuse treatment, and that they can retain this information and can make a free decision. Any patient thought to be lacking the capacity to consent can be treated under the common law.

Common law imposes a duty of care on all professional staff to all persons within the hospital. An individual undertakes to provide proper care to those needing it when taking up a professional appointment in a hospital; hence you as a doctor must act in the best interests of the patient.

The Mental Health Act 1983

> 🔑 The Mental Health Act (MHA) does not apply to the treatment of physical illness.

The MHA allows for the legal detention and treatment of adults with mental illness, mental impairment and psychopathic disorder where their admission and/or treatment are considered necessary in the interests of health and safety, for the protection of others and where they are unable to consent to admission and/or treatment.

The MHA does not apply to the treatment of physical illness, which requires either informed consent from the individual or treatment under common law. The issues can become difficult when physical illness may have led to a disability of the mind through disordered brain function: this area is not always clear-cut. The senior doctor in the department must be involved and a referral made to the psychiatric team as urgently as possible whenever there is consideration of the MHA being used. Any use of the MHA will inevitably take time – for arrival of the appropriate personnel and for their subsequent assessment – so usually the detention of the patient will be under common law.

Section 136

Section 136 of the MHA empowers a police officer to detain and take to a place of safety an individual who may require assessment and/or treatment. In many areas the designated place of safety is a police cell, but some hospital emergency departments may be so designated, although most are ill equipped to deal with disturbed individuals (and should resist taking on this role if they do not have adequate facilities). However, the police will bring any person to the emergency department if they consider that the individual might be medically unfit.

Medical/psychiatric causes of violence and aggression

- Acute confusional state: an acute, transient, fluctuating, potentially reversible, organic brain disorder characterised by globally impaired consciousness and inattention.
- Psychiatric conditions: most commonly personality disorder and substance abuse.
- Other organic brain pathologies.

History of the presenting problem

Dealing with a patient who could be dangerous

- Remember that you have a duty to yourself and other staff members as well as the patient: *do not take risks*.
- *Be safe*: do not see this man on your own; if you meet him in a room (rather than an open area) make sure that he is away from the door and that you are close to the door; if you are wearing a tie, remove it.

The circumstances mean that it will clearly not be possible to get a reliable and useful medical history from the patient. Use any other sources of information that may be available, as described in Section 1.2.31, with points of particular importance being the speed of onset of symptoms, drug or alcohol ingestion/withdrawal, recent history of head trauma, associated symptoms (including headache, seizures and vomiting) and a history of significant past or current medical illness.

Examination and investigation

As with history-taking, it will not be possible to perform a physical examination and pursue investigation in the usual manner if the patient is not cooperative. Try and glean as much information as you can from the following.

- Inspection: are there any signs of trauma, particularly to the head? Are there any localising neurological signs, eg is the patient moving both arms in the same sort of way? Are there any other features that suggest significant medical illness, eg rash?
- Vital signs: if the patient will allow these to be checked. Fever and/or

hypotension are not features of psychiatric illness.

If possible, check fingerprick blood glucose. Other investigation will be determined by clinical suspicion and the willingness (or otherwise) of the patient to cooperate; urine toxicology may be helpful.

Write notes that clearly describe the situation

Your notes in the medical record must give a clear and precise description of the situation. Do not use vague terms such as 'patient uncooperative'. What did he say? Write it down in quotes: 'Patient said "Piss off . . . go away" '. How did he appear: 'Bleeding from head wound and agitated; shouting out loud, sweating, shaking and tremulous; and holding onto a chair and threatening to use it as a weapon'.

Management

If patients are hypoglycaemic (blood glucose <2.5 mmol/L), try to encourage them to drink or eat something sweet, but do not give them a hot drink which they might spill over themselves or throw over you. Obtaining intravenous access is not likely to be straightforward: give glucagon 1 mg im if parenteral treatment is required.

If the patient has another specific medical or surgical diagnosis, then this will require appropriate treatment, but before such treatment can be administered it will be necessary to have a practical strategy for dealing with violence or aggression.

De-escalation techniques

Try to keep calm. Introduce yourself and reassure the patient: speak clearly, do not shout, minimise eye contact and always maintain a safe distance. Ask the patient what the problem is: acknowledge his or her feelings and empathise as appropriate; try to establish an emotional relationship ('I'm trying to help'); and attempt to address any immediate problems or explain why you cannot do so.

Sedation

If the patient needs further assessment or treatment and is not calmed by discussion, then sedation may be required. The synergistic use of an antipsychotic and a benzodiazepine is widely recommended, the benzodiazepine reducing the dose of antipsychotic necessary to produce calm and therefore limiting the risk of oversedation and other side effects. The most desirable end-point of using sedatives in the context of agitation is a calm and cooperative patient not an unresponsive one, which is sometimes a difficult balance to achieve.

Sedation of the violent or aggressive patient

The physician administering sedation must be confident in airway management, have appropriate back-up from the intensive care unit and must also have the correct doses of antagonists available.

Perform sedation as follows.

- Step 1: begin by encouraging the patient to take oral sedation. The oral route is the safest but with the requirement for patient cooperation; the downside is that oral medications take some time to be absorbed. Try lorazepam 1–4 mg stat and haloperidol 2.5 mg stat (rising to 5–10 mg if needed).

- Step 2: give intramuscular sedation. However, be careful to avoid accidental needle-stick injury of individuals other than the patient and remember that the absorption profile of drugs given intramuscularly is also unpredictable. Try lorazepam 1–4 mg stat and haloperidol 2.5 mg stat (rising to 5–10 mg if needed).

- Step 3: if the patient is *in extremis* and you think it essential to induce sedation immediately, request four people trained in control and restraint (one for each arm and one for each leg); request an anaesthetist and ensure that resuscitation equipment is available; and draw up several syringes, each containing a reasonable dose of intravenous benzodiazepine (eg lorazepam 4 mg). When all are assembled, restrain the patient, insert intravenous cannula, inject

one syringe of benzodiazepine, wait 60 seconds and then repeat as necessary until sedation is achieved.

Do not take risks!

If you are confronted with a violent or aggressive patient and genuinely fear for your safety, keep yourself and others out of the patient's way until adequate help is available. Let the patient leave the hospital if trying to do so, informing duty hospital manager and/or police as appropriate.

Where should the violent or aggressive patient be managed?

- If an underlying medical problem requiring admission for treatment is present, admit the patient to a medical ward *when appropriate psychiatric input has been organised*, eg one-to-one psychiatrically trained nurse in attendance.
- If the patient has a psychiatric disorder but no medical disorder, it is up to a psychiatrist to decide if admission to a psychiatric unit is required: *the patient is not to be admitted to a medical ward under any circumstances*.
- If the patient has no underlying psychiatric or medical disorder, *the person should not remain in hospital*; the police should deal with any violent behaviour.

2.1 Overdoses

The general clinical approach to the patient who has taken an overdose is described in Section 1.2.36, to the patient who is in circulatory shock in Section 1.2.2 and to the patient in coma in Section 1.2.31.

 For any patient who has taken an overdose seek advice sooner rather than later from Toxbase on http://www.spib.axl.co.uk/ (this website requires hospital registration to access the service) or phone the National Poisons Information Service (NPIS), who offer a 24-hour telephone information line. For contact details see their website (http://www.npis.org/).

2.1.1 Prevention of drug absorption from the gut

Activated charcoal

This is the preferred method of gut decontamination if the dose of toxin taken is likely to cause moderate to severe toxicity. The single dose (50 g for adults) can be given up to 1 hour after ingestion, but note that some drugs do not readily adsorb to charcoal and that repeated doses may be useful for some toxins (Table 25).

> ⚠️ Charcoal is dangerous if aspirated.

Other techniques

Gastric lavage and/or emetics are now not used, studies having shown that they do not improve clinical outcome; they are definitely contraindicated in any patient who is unable to maintain the airway or following the ingestion of corrosives or organic solvents.

Whole-bowel irrigation with polyethylene glycol solution, given orally or through a nasogastric tube until clear fluid appears per rectum, can be used following ingestion of slow-release preparations (lithium, iron, arsenic, lead oxide and zinc sulphate). However, it is contraindicated if there is an inability to maintain the airway and ileus, or if there is bowel obstruction or haemodynamic instability.

2.1.2 Management of overdoses of specific drugs

Paracetamol

Patients presenting with paracetamol overdose will usually have no symptoms related to paracetamol toxicity. Nausea and vomiting may occur, and right subcostal pain and tenderness suggest hepatic necrosis. The feared complication is acute liver failure, which may develop over days.

> • The plasma paracetamol concentration should be checked in patients suspected of having taken an overdose, at 4 hours post ingestion if they present earlier.
> • Start *N*-acetylcysteine in any patient admitted with paracetamol overdose while awaiting measurement of the paracetamol concentration; stop treatment if the level is non-toxic (Fig. 43).
> • An accurate history is essential for the interpretation of the plasma paracetamol concentration. If there is any doubt, then *N*-acetylcysteine should be given regardless of the level.

Patients sometimes present with toxicologically trivial (but perhaps psychiatrically very significant) overdoses of paracetamol. As a rough guide, paracetamol levels

TABLE 25 USE OF ACTIVATED CHARCOAL AFTER OVERDOSE	
Toxins not adsorbed by charcoal	**Toxins for which repeated doses of charcoal may be useful**
Iron salts	Slow-release preparations
Lithium	Carbamazepine
Ethanol/methanol/ethylene glycol	Dapsone
Acids/alkalis	Digoxin
Organic solvents	Paraquat
Mercury	Phenobarbital
Lead	Quinine
Fluorides	*Amanita phalloides* (death cap mushroom)
Potassium salts	

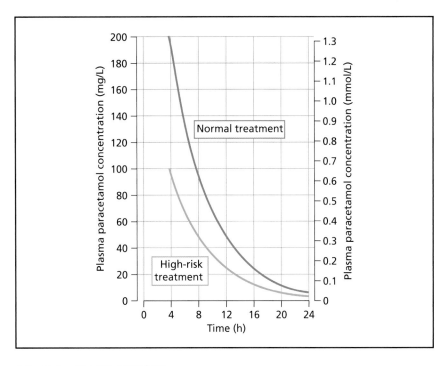

▲ Fig. 43 Paracetamol treatment lines.

Following paracetamol overdose specialist advice from a liver centre should be sought in the presence of any of the following indicators of severe hepatotoxicity.

- INR >2 at 24 hours post ingestion, >4 at 48 hours or >6 at 72 hours.
- PT in seconds is greater than the number of hours since overdose.
- Plasma creatinine >200 μmol/L.
- Hypoglycaemia.
- Acidosis or hypotension (mean arterial pressure <60 mmHg) despite adequate resuscitation.
- Encephalopathy.

are likely to be above the treatment line if more than 150 mg/kg or 12 g, whichever is the smaller, has been taken (>75 mg/kg if the patient is at high risk of toxicity).

Patients at high risk of toxicity following paracetamol overdose

- Patients on enzyme-inducing drugs (eg carbamazepine, phenytoin, rifampicin or phenobarbital) or who are malnourished (owing to anorexia or HIV).
- Patients who drink more than 21 units of alcohol per week if male, or more than 14 units per week if female, may also be at greater risk.

Chronic or staggered paracetamol overdose

In this circumstance the plasma paracetamol concentration cannot be interpreted: if the total dose in 24 hours exceeds 150 mg/kg or 12 g, whichever is the smaller (>75 mg/kg in high-risk patients), then *N*-acetylcysteine should be given.

The dose of *N*-acetylcysteine is 150 mg/kg in 200 mL 5% dextrose intravenously over 15 minutes; then 50 mg/kg in 500 mL 5% dextrose over 4 hours; and then 100 mg/kg in 1000 mL 5% dextrose over 16 hours. Continued *N*-acetylcysteine should be given at a rate of 150 mg/kg over 24 hours if the patient is symptomatic and/or there are abnormalities on investigation, ie raised prothrombin time (PT)/INR and/or elevated plasma creatinine and/or acidosis.

Adverse reactions to *N*-acetylcysteine include nausea, flushing, urticaria, angio-oedema, bronchospasm and hypotension. These usually occur early and often resolve if *N*-acetylcysteine is stopped and intravenous chlorpheniramine given, after which the infusion may be restarted at the lowest rate. Methionine 2.5 g orally can be given to those who are intolerant of *N*-acetylcysteine and is protective if given within 12 hours.

Tricyclic antidepressants

Coma, convulsions and arrhythmias are the most serious signs of toxicity. Tachycardia and QRS prolongation (>100 ms) on ECG indicate severe poisoning. Anticholinergic effects include blurred vision, dry mouth, pupillary dilation and urinary retention. Central effects include confusion, drowsiness, nystagmus, ataxia, hyperreflexia and hyperthermia.

The most important aspects of management are cardiac monitoring and efforts to increase urinary excretion of the tricyclic by alkaline diuresis.

- Place on cardiac monitor: dysrhythmias may respond to correction of hypoxia and acidosis, but antiarrhythmic drugs may be necessary, although some can exacerbate the toxic effects of tricyclics (seek expert advice).

- Urinary alkalinisation with sodium bicarbonate is indicated if there is systemic acidosis, prolonged QRS, ventricular arrhythmias, hypotension or cardiac arrest. Infuse sodium chloride 0.9% 250 mL/hour iv to induce diuresis of >150 mL/hour. When diuresis is established check urinary pH and replace saline with sodium bicarbonate 1.26% (500 mL over 2 hours) if it is necessary to obtain urinary pH between 7.45 and 7.55. When a satisfactory urinary pH is attained, replace sodium bicarbonate with saline. Continue to monitor urinary pH and give further bicarbonate if urinary pH falls significantly.

- Give intravenous benzodiazepine for convulsions.

Salicylates

The important clinical features are hyperventilation, tinnitus, deafness, sweating, vasodilatation, convulsions, coma and death.

Important aspects of management include checking arterial blood gases: respiratory alkalosis and/or metabolic acidosis can be expected. If salicylate levels are >500 mg/L (3.6 mmol/L), consider alkaline diuresis with 1.26% sodium bicarbonate (as described above for tricyclic overdose); if salicylate levels are >700 mg/L (5.1 mmol/L), consider haemodialysis.

3.1 Central venous lines

3.1.1 Indications, contraindications, consent and preparation

Indications for insertion of a central line

These include the infusion of fluids (including parenteral feeding), infusion of drugs (eg inotropes and hypertonic solutions), measurement of central venous pressure, insertion of a temporary pacing wire and access for haemodialysis/haemofiltration.

Contraindications to insertion of a central line

There are no absolute contraindications, but relative contraindications include the following.

- Abnormal clotting.

- Marked hypovolaemia: the technique is difficult, time-consuming and carries more risk of complications, so it is always best to correct hypovolaemia through large-bore peripheral or femoral vein access before inserting a central vein cannula.

- Severe respiratory disease: a relative contraindication for the subclavian approach because a pneumothorax may precipitate respiratory failure.

- Local sepsis.

Consent for insertion of a central line

Whether verbal or written consent for central line insertion should be obtained from the patient will depend on the clinical context. If central lines are being inserted in the non-emergency situation, then written consent will be required in most hospitals, and many will have specific consent forms for the purpose. The broad principles of informed consent apply: patients need to know and understand the indication for the procedure; the details of the procedure, including the need to lie still and (relatively) flat; and the potential complications (Table 26).

Preparation for central line insertion

Check platelet count and clotting, and obtain informed consent. Ensure adequate monitoring is available (ECG and pulse oximeter). Prepare equipment as follows:

- dressing pack, drapes and gloves (all sterile);

- local anaesthetic, syringe and needle;

- Seldinger catheter set with 5-mL syringe, introducer needle, guidewire, dilator and central line, or a 16G long cannula;

- saline or Hepsal flush;

- three-way tap (×3 if triple-lumen catheter);

- small scalpel blade, silk suture and sterile occlusive dressing.

Technique for central line insertion

The National Institute for Health and Clinical Excellence (NICE) guidelines allow operators experienced in the landmark technique to continue to use it: junior medical staff should learn to use ultrasound to identify and cannulate the vessel.

TABLE 26 COMPLICATIONS ARISING FROM CENTRAL LINE INSERTION[1]

Frequency	Internal jugular	Subclavian
Common	Arterial puncture (2–8%) Pneumothorax (<1%) Bruising/haematoma formation Infection	Arterial puncture (2–4%) Pneumothorax/haemopneumothorax (1–2.5%) Bruising/haematoma formation Infection
Less common/rare	Nerve damage Arteriovenous fistula Venous thrombosis Lost catheters	Nerve damage Chylothorax (especially left-sided lines) Arteriovenous fistula Venous thrombosis Lost catheters

1. It is not sensible to inform patients of every possible complication that might arise from central line insertion (or any other procedure). However, in the context of explaining the indications and potential benefits to them of the procedure, it would be expected that they would be told of the common problems that can arise.

3.1.2 Specific techniques for insertion of central lines

Internal jugular vein cannulation using the Seldinger technique

- Ask the the patient to lie down, preferably with a head-down tilt, and turn the head away from the side you intend to cannulate.

- Identify your landmarks (Fig. 44): the internal jugular vein lies superficial, lateral and parallel to the carotid artery. Identify the apex of the triangle formed by the two heads of the sternocleidomastoid muscle at the level of the thyroid cartilage. This is where you will introduce the needle, one of the so-called 'high approaches' that minimise the risk of pneumothorax.

- Clean and drape the skin.

- Infiltrate the skin and subcutaneous tissue with 1% lidocaine (lignocaine).

- Flush the lumen(s) of the central line with saline or Hepsal and ensure you have all your equipment within easy reach.

- Attach the introducer needle to the 5-mL syringe and, keeping one finger on the carotid pulse, insert the needle just lateral to this at 45° to the skin. Aim for the ipsilateral nipple in men or the anterior superior iliac spine in women. Advance the needle slowly whilst aspirating for blood. You will only need to insert it a few centimetres as the vein lies superficially. If you do not hit the vein, withdraw the needle to just below the skin and aim slightly more medially and superficially before trying again.

- Once you are in the vein and can aspirate blood freely, remove the syringe and occlude the end of the needle with your finger (to prevent air embolism).

Seldinger technique

This technique, which is more reliable than cannula-over-needle techniques, is widely used for arterial or venous cannulation.

- Once you are in the vein and can aspirate blood freely, remove the syringe and occlude the end of the needle with your finger to prevent air embolism.

- Pass the guidewire into the vein, ensuring that it passes freely. Remove the wire if there is any resistance and check that blood can still be aspirated easily, then try again.

- Remove the needle, leaving the wire in the vein.

- Nick the skin at the base of the wire with the small scalpel blade to allow easy passage of the dilator. If there is resistance do not use force, which can crimp the guidewire or the end of the dilator. The usual explanation is that an inadequate nick has been made with the scalpel blade.

- Pass the dilator over the wire through the subcutaneous tissue and then remove it, leaving the wire *in situ*.

- Pass the central line over the wire into the vein.

- Remove the wire and check that you can aspirate blood freely through the cannula.

- With the line in place, flush with saline or Hepsal and close the line off to air.

- Secure with a suture and place a sterile occlusive dressing over the site.

If measurement of the central venous pressure (CVP) is needed, attach the manometer set to the patient and adjust the zero reference point on the manometer so it is at the level of the patient's right atrium (mid-axillary line). Alternatively, an electronic transducer and oscilloscope may be used to continuously measure the CVP, which also need to be zeroed and calibrated prior to use.

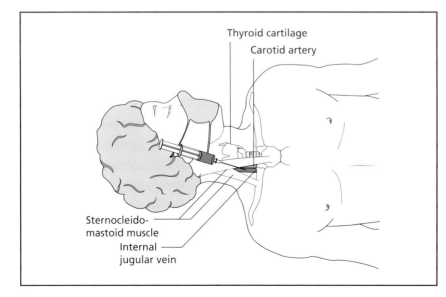

Thyroid cartilage
Carotid artery
Sternocleido-mastoid muscle
Internal jugular vein

▲ **Fig. 44** Cannulation of the internal jugular vein.

Subclavian vein cannulation using the Seldinger technique

The axillary vein becomes the subclavian vein at the lateral border of the first rib and extends for 3–4 cm, just deep to the clavicle. It forms the brachiocephalic vein with the internal jugular vein behind the sternoclavicular joint. The right subclavian vein is easier to cannulate than the left. Cannulation is as follows.

- Identify the landmarks (Fig. 45): locate the suprasternal notch, sternoclavicular joint and acromioclavicular joint and select a point one finger-breadth below the junction of the medial third and middle third of the clavicle.

- Clean and drape the skin.

- Infiltrate the skin and subcutaneous tissue with 1% lidocaine (lignocaine).

- Flush the lumen(s) of the central line with saline or Hepsal and ensure you have all your equipment within easy reach.

- Insert the introducer needle attached to the 5-mL syringe until it hits the clavicle and 'walk' the tip down the clavicle until

it is lying just under the inferior border. Advance the needle, aspirating for blood, towards the contralateral sternoclavicular joint. Try to keep the track of the needle parallel to the bed in order to avoid puncturing the pleura or subclavian artery.

- Once blood is aspirated freely, rotate the bevel of the needle towards the heart in order to maximise the chance of the wire passing down the brachiocephalic vein rather than up the internal jugular vein.

- Insert the central line using the Seldinger technique.

After the procedure arrange a CXR to exclude a pneumothorax and to confirm the correct position of the catheter: ideally the tip should lie in the superior vena cava just above the right atrium.

Femoral vein cannulation using the Seldinger technique

- Identify your landmarks (Fig. 46): the femoral vein lies directly medial to the femoral artery in the femoral triangle (as remembered by the acronym 'NAVY': nerve, artery, vein and Y-fronts).

- Clean and drape the skin.

- Infiltrate the skin and subcutaneous tissue with 1% lidocaine (lignocaine).

- Flush the lumen(s) of the central line with saline or Hepsal and ensure you have all your equipment within easy reach.

- Feel the femoral pulse and insert the introducer needle one finger-breadth medial to this, angulating it slightly towards the patient's head, but keeping it in line with the long axis of the leg. Advance slowly, aspirating all the time until there is free flow of blood into the syringe.

- Insert the central line using the Seldinger technique.

- With the line in place, flush with saline or Hepsal and close the line off to air. Secure with a suture and place a sterile occlusive dressing over the site.

> ⚠ **Do not make a bad situation worse**
>
> - If the carotid artery is punctured and a haematoma forms, do not attempt internal jugular vein cannulation on the other side (especially in patients with abnormal clotting): bilateral haematomas may result in airway compromise. Cannulate the subclavian or femoral vein instead.
> - Do not attempt to cannulate the opposite subclavian vessel if the first attempt was unsuccessful: giving a patient bilateral pneumothoraces is not recommended. Do a check CXR or cannulate the internal jugular or femoral vein instead.
> - In ventilated patients even a small pneumothorax must be treated with a chest drain as it may rapidly develop into a tension pneumothorax.

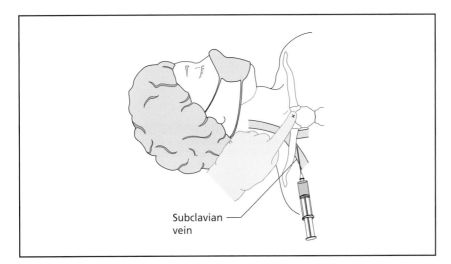

Subclavian vein

▲**Fig. 45** Cannulation of the subclavian vein.

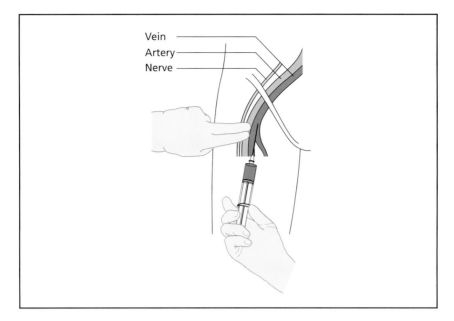

▲ **Fig. 46** Cannulation of the femoral vein.

3.1.3 Interpretation of central venous pressure measurements

Before measuring the central venous pressure (CVP) ensure that the system has been zeroed to the mid-axillary reference point and that the venous pressure swings with respiration.

The CVP gives an indication of the patient's blood volume but is also affected by the contractile state of the myocardium, venous tone, intrathoracic pressure and pulmonary arterial pressure. It does not always provide accurate information on left-sided cardiac filling pressures, which can be low even though the CVP is normal or high, the classic example of this being severe pulmonary embolism (PE).

The normal range for the CVP is $3–8$ cmH$_2$O (blood) if zero is defined as 5 cm below the angle of Louis

(sometimes incorrectly called the 'method of Louis') or $7–12$ cmH$_2$O if zero is defined according to the phlebostatic axis (the mid-point between the anterior and posterior surfaces of the chest at the level of the fourth intercostal space). Causes of an abnormal CVP are shown in Table 27.

3.2 Lumbar puncture

Indications for performing a lumbar puncture

- Diagnostic indications are meningitis, subarachnoid haemorrhage and intrathecal malignancy;

- Therapeutic indications are intrathecal drug administration and benign intracranial hypertension.

Contraindications to performing a lumbar puncture

These include raised intracranial pressure, posterior fossa or spinal cord mass lesions, local sepsis, and a bleeding tendency.

Lumbar puncture and risk of coning

If a patient is unconscious, drowsy or has clinical features of raised intracranial pressure or focal neurological signs, then a CT scan must be performed prior to lumbar puncture. Antibiotic treatment should be started immediately if there is likely to be a delay and meningitis is a diagnostic possibility.

TABLE 27 CAUSES OF AN ABNORMAL CVP		
CVP reading	**Real or artefact?**	**Cause**
High	Genuine	Fluid overload
		Right ventricular failure, eg right ventricular infarction
		Massive PE
		Cardiac tamponade
		Tension pneumothorax
	Error	Incorrect zero
		Incorrect placement: catheter tip in right ventricle will give an unexpectedly high pressure
		Blocked catheter: causes a sustained high reading with a damped waveform
		Infusion of fluid, eg through an infusion pump, at the same time as the pressure is being measured
Low	Genuine	Hypovolaemia
		Septic shock
		Anaphylactic shock
	Error	Incorrect zero

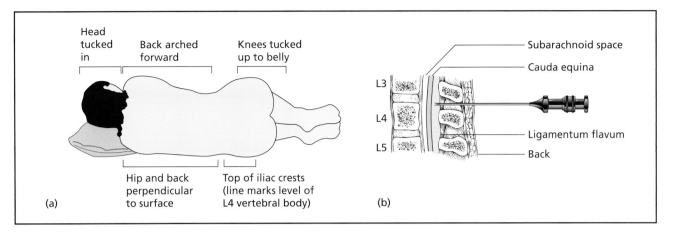

▲ **Fig. 47** Technique for lumbar puncture. (**a**) The patient should be curled up to increase the space between the vertebrae. (**b**) The needle should be advanced slowly until it penetrates the ligamentum flavum: a flashback of CSF when the stylet is removed indicates correct positioning.

Preparation

Check platelet count and clotting, and obtain informed consent. Prepare equipment as follows:

- dressing pack, gown, drapes and gloves (all sterile);

- local anaesthetic, syringe and needles;

- antiseptic;

- lumbar puncture needles and sterile manometer;

- sample tubes (serum glucose bottle and sterile 20-mL containers for differential counts, bacteriology and protein estimation).

Technique

- Ask the patient to lie on the bed (Fig. 47a). Positioning is all-important: the knees should be drawn up towards the chest to open the space between the spinous processes, and the spine should be parallel to the bed.

- Gown and glove up.

- Prepare the skin with antiseptic and cover with sterile drapes.

- Locate the puncture site (L3/4 or L4/5).

- Anaesthetise the skin and subcutaneous tissues with 5–10 mL 1% lidocaine (lignocaine) using a 25G needle; then switch to an 18G needle and infiltrate the deeper tissues.

- Assemble the manometer and unscrew the tops of the sterile containers.

- Insert the lumbar puncture needle at 90° to the skin: advance slowly, aiming between two spinous processes. There is a slight loss of resistance as the needle enters the dural space (Fig. 47b).

- Remove the stylet and ensure that cerebrospinal fluid (CSF) drips freely from the needle. If no CSF is forthcoming, insert the stylet and advance the needle a few millimetres and check again.

- Attach the manometer and measure the pressure (normal 6–15 cmH$_2$O).

- Collect CSF samples: 2–5 drops for biochemistry; 5–10 drops for bacteriology (ask for urgent microscopy and Gram stain, and culture, sensitivities and viral studies); and 5–10 drops for cytology.

- Remove the needle and dress the wound.

- Ask the patient to remain lying flat for 2–4 hours to reduce the severity of post-lumbar puncture headache.

Always send blood samples for glucose and protein estimation at the same time as CSF samples: the CSF glucose concentration is normally 60–80% of the blood level. In cases of suspected subarachnoid haemorrhage (SAH), the red cell count in consecutive samples can help to distinguish SAH from a bloody tap, and the samples should also be examined for xanthochromia (oxyhaemoglobin and bilirubin).

Normal values and values in disease for CSF pressure, cell counts, glucose concentration and protein concentration are shown in Table 28.

3.3 Cardiac pacing

There are three common types of cardiac pacing: transvenous endocardial (may be temporary or permanent), epicardial (in

TABLE 28 CSF FINDINGS IN VARIOUS CONDITIONS

	Pressure (cmH$_2$O)	White cells (per µL)	Protein (g/L)	Glucose (mmol/L)
Normal	6–15	≤5 Mononuclear cells	0.2–0.4	2.5–4.5
Bacterial meningitis	Normal or ↑	↑↑↑ Polymorphs	1–5	0.2–2.2
Viral meningitis	Normal or ↑	↑ to ↑↑ Lymphocytes	≤1	Normal
Tumour	Normal or ↑	0–100s Mononuclear cells Malignant cells also possible	↑↑	Normal or ↓

association with cardiac surgery) and transcutaneous/external.

Common indications for pacing

Bradyarrhythmias
Temporary pacing The decision to pace is based on the presence of haemodynamic compromise or potential to do so rather than the specific rhythm.

- Patients with second- or third-degree atrioventricular (AV) block may need temporary pacing prior to general anaesthesia.

- Patients with second- or third-degree heart block in association with an acute myocardial infarction may require pacing (this may be complicated by the need to obtain central venous access in someone who has received thrombolysis).

Permanent pacing There are two types of indication for permanent pacing, class 1 and class 2.

- Class 1 indications: chronic symptomatic second- or third-degree AV block, and sinoatrial node dysfunction with recurrent syncope.

- Class 2 indications: asymptomatic third-degree AV block and resistant sinus bradycardia.

Tachyarrhythmias
Some tachyarrhythmias (AV nodal re-entrant tachycardia, AV re-entry tachycardia, atrial flutter and ventricular tachycardia) may be treated by pacing or by premature electrical stimulation. This may be done by a temporary transvenous pacing wire or, if persistent, by a permanent system.

Technique for external pacing
After explaining to the patient what you are going to do and ensuring adequate sedation/analgesia, follow the procedure below.

- Place one electrode in a position equivalent to lead V2–V3 of the ECG, with the other either over the apex of the heart or on the posterior of the chest below the left scapula (Fig. 48).

- Set the pacing box to demand, with a rate of approximately 60 bpm.

- Connect the leads to the patient and slowly increase the current; 50–100 mA is usually required.

- Ventricular capture is indicated when a pacing spike is associated with a ventricular complex and a palpable pulse wave.

- Make immediate arrangements for transvenous pacing: external pacing is unreliable and should be continued for as short a period as possible.

If external pacing is unsuccessful ensure there is adequate current, then try other electrodes or electrode positions, percussion pacing (forceful rhythmic thumping of the left anterior chest), isoprenaline infusion, or immediate transvenous pacing.

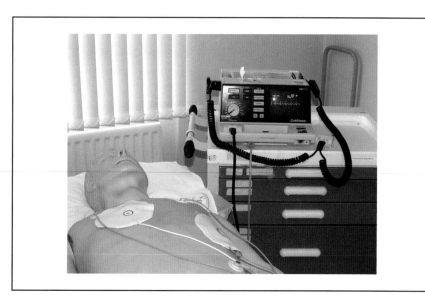

▲ **Fig. 48** External pacing with a modern monitor/defibrillator/external pacer.

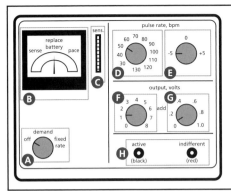

A Mode: demand vs fixed

B Pointer: allows you to see whether an intrinsic beat is sensed or if the patient is being paced

C Sensitivity should be set at 1.0

D Rate setting

E Rate adjustment by ± 5 bpm

F & G Voltage adjustment: should be set at 2 volts above threshold

H Lead terminals

▲**Fig. 49** A common type of pacemaker generator.

Common problems of transvenous pacing

The procedure for temporary transvenous pacing is beyond the scope of this module, but it is important for all doctors working on hospital wards to be aware of the common problems that can arise with transvenous pacing once it has been established.

- Increasing threshold: temporary transvenous pacemakers should have their threshold tested at least daily as this often increases over time. Testing is done by gradually turning down the pacemaker current until failure to capture occurs. The pacemaker output should be set at three times the threshold voltage or 3 V, whichever is the higher. Increasing threshold is an indication for repositioning of the wire or urgent permanent pacing (Fig. 49).

- Loss of electrical continuity: the commonest reason for sudden failure of a pacemaker to work, which may result in symptomatic bradycardia, is a loose connection. There are generally four connections between the pacing electrodes and the pacemaker box: check them all.

- Electrode displacement: the tip of the transvenous pacemaker should be in the right ventricle; migration

of the pacing wire can lead to an increasing threshold or sudden bradycardia.

> 🔑 If a temporary pacemaker suddenly stops working, always check the connections before you do anything else.

3.4 Elective DC cardioversion

Indication and preparation

The indication for elective DC cardioversion is tachyarrhythmias causing cardiovascular compromise, significant symptoms or symptoms that are resistant to drug therapy.

Consider anticoagulation: cardioversion of atrial fibrillation has a thromboembolic risk of around 5%, so patients should be therapeutically anticoagulated with warfarin for 6 weeks before elective cardioversion for this indication.

Check the electrolytes and ensure that digoxin toxicity has been excluded.

Technique

After obtaining consent from the patient, who should be starved in

case of the need for intubation, proceed as follows.

- Ensure there is adequate intravenous access.

- Ensure there is adequate monitoring and that a defibrillator is available: ECG electrodes must be applied to the chest and connected to the defibrillator.

- Ensure the availability of emergency drugs.

- Ensure there is adequate sedation/analgesia: experienced personnel may perform elective cardioversion under sedation alone; many prefer general anaesthesia.

- Apply gel pads to position V2–V3 on the anterior chest and over the apex of the heart.

- Ensure the defibrillator is set to apply a synchronised shock.

- Charge the defibrillator while the paddles are applied to the patient's chest. Appropriate starting voltages depend on the arrhythmia: atrial fibrillation, 200 J (120–150 J biphasic); atrial flutter, 100 J (70–120 J biphasic); supraventricular tachycardia, 100 J (70–120 J biphasic); ventricular tachycardia, 200 J (120–150 J biphasic).

- Discharge the current only after ensuring that it is safe to do so.

- Recheck the cardiac rhythm and the patient's observations.

3.5 Intercostal chest drain insertion

Indications

- Pneumothorax: in any ventilated patient; tension pneumothorax after initial needle thoracocentesis; persistent or recurrent pneumothorax after simple aspiration; large secondary spontaneous pneumothorax in patients aged over 50 years.

- Malignant pleural effusion.

- Empyema and complicated parapneumonic pleural effusion.

- Traumatic haemopneumothorax.

- Postoperative, eg thoracotomy, oesophagectomy and cardiac surgery.

Small-bore chest drains (10–14Fr) are recommended: they are as effective as large-bore tubes in most circumstances and are better tolerated by the patient. Large-bore tubes (28–32Fr) should be used for haemothoraces and in the event of failure to drain a pneumothorax via a small-bore tube. They may also still have a role in the treatment of empyema, although increasing success is being seen with small-bore drains in conjunction with thrombolytic therapy.

> ⚠️ **Tension pneumothorax**
>
> Never wait for a CXR if a tension pneumothorax has been diagnosed on clinical grounds: do an immediate needle thoracocentesis and then insert a chest drain (see Section 1.2.14).

Preparation

> ⚠️ Begin by careful radiological assessment: you do not want to insert a drain into an emphysematous bulla by mistake.

- Risk assessment: coagulopathy or platelet deficit should be corrected prior to chest drain insertion. If

the patient is on warfarin this should be stopped, aiming for an INR <1.5 prior to the procedure unless he/she has a prosthetic heart valve, in which case advice should be sought.

- Explain the benefits, risks and technique of the procedure and obtain patient consent.

- Intravenous access: this should be established in all patients. If the procedure is being done for a haemothorax, ensure that you have two large-bore intravenous cannulae in place and blood available for transfusion before starting the procedure.

- Monitoring: the patient should be on oxygen during the procedure, with monitoring of oxygen saturation throughout.

- Premedication: this should be considered and offered to every patient who is not *in extremis*, eg midazolam (1–5 mg iv).

- Equipment. Make sure you have everything you need on the trolley before you start: basic sterile pack; local anaesthetic and syringes with orange and green needles; chest drain insertion pack (Fig. 50)

complete with chest drain (and connectors), guidewire and dilators (replaced by Spencer Wells forceps if it is a large-bore drain), scalpel and handle, syringe and needle; scissors; suture 1/0 or 2/0 silk; dressings; and an underwater seal bottle with connections.

Technique

- Position the patient, ideally in a semi-recumbent position with hand resting behind the head.

- Identify the landmarks (Fig. 51): the safest position for chest drain insertion is in the fifth intercostal space in the mid-axillary line. In a patient without large breasts this will be at the level of the nipple; in someone with large breasts select the intercostal space a hand's width below the axilla.

- Clean and drape the skin: aseptic technique should be observed at all times.

- Infiltrate the skin with local anaesthetic using the orange needle and then infiltrate down to the pleura using the green needle; then go through the pleura to aspirate air or fluid.

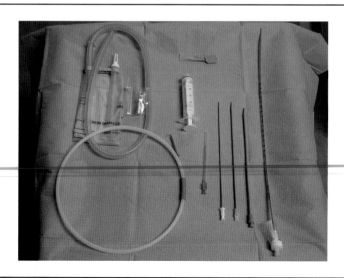

▲ **Fig. 50** Chest drain insertion pack.

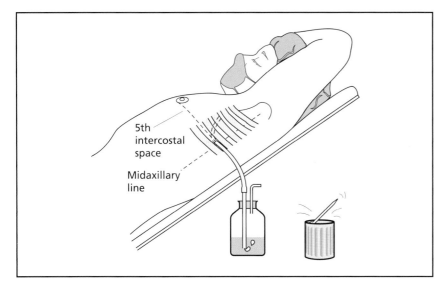

5th intercostal space

Midaxillary line

▲ **Fig. 51** Landmarks for insertion of an intercostal chest drain.

> ⚠ A chest drain should not be inserted if free air or fluid cannot be aspirated with a needle at the time of introduction of local anaesthesia. Obtain further image guidance.

Small-bore chest drain insertion using Seldinger technique

- Insert the supplied needle into the pleural space, ensuring you aspirate to reconfirm position.

- Pass the guidewire through the needle and then carefully withdraw the needle leaving the guidewire *in situ*.

- Pass the dilator over the guidewire and through the subcutaneous tissue into the pleural space. A small incision in the skin and subcutaneous tissue may be necessary prior to dilator insertion. Withdraw the dilator, leaving the guidewire *in situ*.

- Pass the chest drain over the guidewire into the pleural space and then withdraw the guidewire.

- Connect the chest drain to an underwater seal and confirm position: oscillation, fluid drainage and bubbling.

- Secure the drain in place with a 1/0 or 2/0 silk suture: tie it so that the skin is closed either side of the drain and then wrap it around and tie it to the drain as many times as its length allows.

- Apply a clear, impervious dressing and ensure the joins between drain and connectors are secured.

> ⚠ You must keep hold of the guidewire at all times when inserting a small-bore chest drain using the Seldinger technique.

Large-bore chest drain insertion

- Make a 2–3 cm incision through the skin and subcutaneous adipose tissue along the line of the intercostal space, just above the edge of the lower rib.

- Bluntly dissect down to the pleura using forceps.

- Puncture the parietal pleura with the tip of the forceps and then insert your finger to enlarge the hole. Sweep your finger around to clear any adhesions or clots. Make sure there is adequate space to insert the drain without using force.

- Remove any trocar from the chest drain and slide the drain over your finger into the thoracic cavity.

- Connect the chest drain to an underwater seal and confirm position: oscillation, fluid drainage and bubbling.

- Secure the drain in place with a 1/0 or 2/0 silk suture: tie it so that the skin is closed either side of the drain and then wrap it around and tie it to the drain as many times as its length allows.

- Apply a clear, impervious dressing and ensure the joins between drain and connectors are secured.

After the procedure

Observe that the drain is functioning: oscillation with respiration, fluid drainage and/or bubbling. Order a CXR to confirm correct positioning of the drain. Prescribe adequate analgesia.

Inform nursing staff of requirements for managing the chest drain:

- never clamp a bubbling chest drain;

- controlled drainage of a large pleural effusion to prevent re-expansion pulmonary oedema;

- accurate recording of fluid drainage and daily function of the chest drain.

Daily assessment of the patient and review of the chest drain is vital. A repeat CXR should be obtained if fluid stops draining, bubbling stops, there is no clear evidence of oscillation of the chest drain or there are concerns with the patient's condition. However, it is not necessary to repeat the CXR daily as a routine.

The chest drain can be removed if there is no fluid drainage or bubbling for >24 hours following radiographic confirmation of resolution of the effusion or pneumothorax. In malignant effusions pleurodesis may be considered prior to removal. The CXR should be repeated following removal of the drain.

> If there is failure of the fluid level to swing with respiration, check the following.
>
> • Is the tube kinked?
> • Is the tube blocked?
> • Is the tube in the wrong position?

> **Causes of a persistent pneumothorax**
>
> • Large primary leak.
> • Leakage at the skin or underwater seal.
> • Bronchopleural fistula.

Complications of inserting a chest drain

- Damage to intrathoracic and/or abdominal organs or vessels: this can be avoided by using the finger sweep and never using the trocar for large-bore chest drain insertion.

- Damage to the intercostal nerve, artery or vein: avoid making the incision below the rib as the intercostal nerves and vessels lie beneath the lower edge of the rib.

- Sepsis (empyema formation or cellulitis): ensure complete aseptic technique, and do not leave chest drains in for longer than necessary.

- Pulmonary oedema if the lung expands rapidly following drainage of a large pleural effusion: drainage of pleural fluid should be limited to around 200 mL/hour.

- Surgical emphysema.

- Haematoma: check that there are no clotting or platelet abnormalities prior to insertion.

- Pain: ensure there is adequate analgesia.

3.6 Arterial blood gases

3.6.1 Measurement of arterial blood gases

Indications for arterial blood gases (ABGs) include pulse oximetry showing Po_2 <92% and any acute unexplained severe illness. There are no absolute contraindications, although severe bleeding disorder is a relative contraindication.

Explain the procedure to the patient (those who have had ABGs performed know just how painful they can be) and then proceed as follows.

Preparation

- Site: choose the site for arterial puncture carefully (radial, brachial or femoral). The radial is most commonly used, in which case first perform the Allen test to check the patency of the ulnar artery: ask the patient to clench the fist firmly, applying pressure to the radial artery, and then ask him or her to relax the fist, at which point the hand should pink up within 10 seconds.

- Equipment: before taking the sample, make sure you know where the blood gas machine is

and how to use it! Assemble alcohol swabs and a preheparinised ABG syringe or a 2-mL syringe into which you have drawn up and then expelled 0.5 mL of heparin solution (5000 units/mL) through an appropriate needle. 25G needles are perfectly adequate for obtaining ABG samples from a radial artery; 18G or 23G are needed for a femoral sample.

Technique

- After gloving up, lay the index and middle fingers of your non-dominant hand along the line of the artery as a guide (Fig. 52).

- For radial and brachial samples hold the syringe at 45–60° to the skin and slowly advance in the line of the artery; for femoral samples hold the syringe at 90° to the skin. There is debate over the use of lidocaine (lignocaine): while this is undoubtedly useful at easing pain if you are unlucky enough to fail first time, its use is painful in itself and it often makes palpation of the artery more difficult.

- A flush of blood indicates puncture of a vessel: with some ABG syringes the arterial pressure will fill the syringe to a predetermined volume; in others you will need to aspirate 1–2 mL.

- Apply pressure to the puncture site for 3 minutes (5 minutes if the patient is anticoagulated).

- Expel all air from the syringe; remove and dispose of the needle and cap the syringe.

- If there is to be a delay in processing the sample, pack it in ice.

- After the procedure check that bleeding has stopped, the main complication being haematoma.

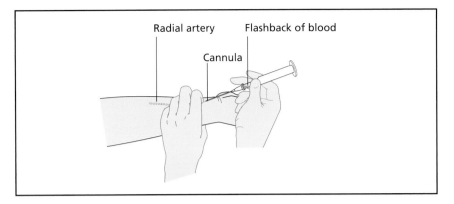

▲**Fig. 52** Taking a sample from the radial artery. The artery should be palpated with two fingers placed along the line of the artery. The needle should be inserted at 45–60° to the skin and slowly advanced in the direction of the artery. A flashback of blood indicates successful puncture.

3.6.2 Interpretation of arterial blood gases

Table 29 shows normal arterial blood gas (ABG) values.

The standard base excess (SBE) is a figure calculated by many blood gas machines as an aid to interpretation of ABG results. The principles of the calculation are as follows.

- Predict the pH that would arise in normal blood in the presence of the $P\text{co}_2$ actually measured. If the $P\text{co}_2$ is high, then the predicted pH is low; if the $P\text{co}_2$ is low, then the predicted pH is high.

- Calculate the amount of acid or base that would have to be added to the blood to change the calculated pH into the pH as actually measured.

- This value is the base deficit or excess (in mmol/L), which quantifies the metabolic

component of acid–base disturbance: the more negative the value of the SBE, the greater the degree of metabolic acidosis.

The types of metabolic and respiratory acid–base disturbances and their common causes are shown in Table 30.

3.7 Airway management

Stridor, gurgling and snoring all suggest an airway at risk. Recognition of airway compromise depends on the following basic and life-saving techniques: look, listen and feel.

- Look for chest movement.

- Listen and feel for air movement at the nose and mouth.

All unconscious patients are at risk.

- A patient with a Glasgow Coma Scale (GCS) score of <8 will need endotracheal intubation unless a cause can be rapidly found and corrected.

- Patients with a GCS score of 8–12 may need basic adjuncts to maintain airway patency.

> Airway compromise results in rapid hypoxia and secondary brain injury. Airway management is the first priority in basic life support (airway, breathing and circulation), but be wary of patients who are spontaneously ventilating but who cannot protect their airway because of a reduction in conscious level.

> Oxygen should be given to all patients with decreased conscious levels unless specifically contraindicated.

3.7.1 Basic airway management

Opening the airway

Head tilt/chin lift
Loss of muscle control leads to occlusion of the airway by the tongue, epiglottis and soft palate. With the patient supine, extend the head on the neck by placing one hand on the forehead and pushing backwards. Place the fingers of the other hand under the tip of the jaw and lift the chin upwards (Fig. 53a).

Jaw thrust
Place the fingers of both hands behind the angles of the mandible. Use upward pressure to lift the jaw forward (Fig. 53b).

TABLE 29 NORMAL ABG VALUES

	Normal range
pH	7.35–7.45
$P\text{co}_2$	4.5–6.0 kPa
Bicarbonate	22–28 mmol/L
Standard base excess	±2 mmol/L
$P\text{o}_2$	10.5–14 kPa (breathing air)
Oxygen saturation	95–100%

TABLE 30 TYPES OF METABOLIC AND RESPIRATORY ACID–BASE DISTURBANCES

Type of disturbance	pH	P_{CO_2}	HCO_3^-	Base excess	Common causes
Metabolic acidosis	Low, or normal if there is respiratory compensation	Low due to secondary respiratory alkalosis	Low: this is the primary abnormality in metabolic acidosis	Negative: this is the base deficit, which quantifies the metabolic component of acid–base disturbances. The more negative the value, the greater the degree of metabolic acidosis	Lactic acidosis: exercise, shock and drugs (metformin) Ketoacidosis: diabetes Hyperchloraemic: bicarbonate wasting, eg renal losses and gastrointestinal fistulae High anion gap: poisoning, eg methanol and antifreeze
Respiratory acidosis	Low, or normal if there has been metabolic compensation	High: primary abnormality is alveolar hypoventilation	Normal in acute respiratory acidosis; high if there has been time for renal compensation	Normal	Acute: bronchopneumonia and severe acute asthma Chronic: chronic obstructive pulmonary disease, neuromuscular disorders and restrictive lung diseases
Respiratory alkalosis	Elevated if acute, normal if there has been metabolic compensation	Low: primary abnormality is alveolar hyperventilation	Normal in acute respiratory alkalosis; low if there has been time for renal compensation	Normal	Anxiety Pain Hypoxia causing stimulation of respiratory centre, eg pulmonary oedema and pneumonia Salicylate overdose: initially causes direct stimulation of the respiratory centre (but also uncouples oxidative phosphorylation leading to metabolic acidosis)
Metabolic alkalosis	Elevated: there is rarely significant respiratory compensation	Usually normal: little, if any, compensatory rise	Elevated: primary abnormality in metabolic alkalosis	Positive: the more positive the value, the greater the degree of metabolic alkalosis	Chronic potassium depletion, eg vomiting and diuretics Chloride loss, eg vomiting

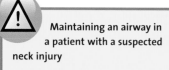

Maintaining an airway in a patient with a suspected neck injury

The jaw thrust method is preferred because it results in less neck movement, but remember that patients with a neck injury are more likely to die from airway obstruction than damage due to neck movement.

Removing obstructions from the oropharynx

Solid foreign material should be removed using Magill forceps or a finger sweep under direct vision. Semi-solid material or liquid should be removed using a Yankauer sucker.

Basic adjuncts to airway control

Oropharyngeal and nasopharyngeal airways help to prevent occlusion of the pharynx by the tongue and soft tissues (Fig. 54). Patients with preserved laryngeal reflexes will generally not tolerate an oropharyngeal airway but may tolerate a nasopharyngeal one.

Insertion of an oropharyngeal airway

Select an airway that corresponds in length to the distance between the corner of the patient's mouth and the angle of the jaw. Open the patient's mouth. Introduce the airway upside down and rotate it 180° as it passes into the oropharynx. Reassess the airway.

Potential problems with oropharyngeal airways

- Incorrect insertion of the airway can exacerbate the problem by pushing the tongue further back.
- In the presence of laryngeal reflexes, insertion of an oropharyngeal airway can trigger vomiting and laryngospasm.

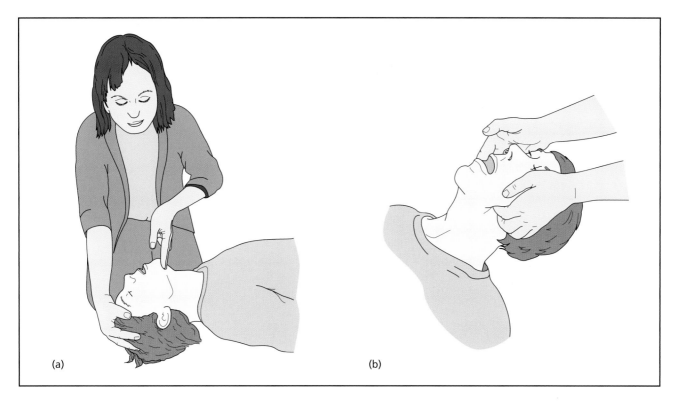

(a)   (b)

▲ **Fig. 53** Opening the airway. (**a**) Head tilt/chin lift method: place one hand on the patient's forehead and the other under the point of the patient's chin, then tilt the head back to open the airway. (**b**) Jaw thrust method: with the index and middle fingers behind the angle of the mandible, apply upward and forward pressure to lift the jaw.

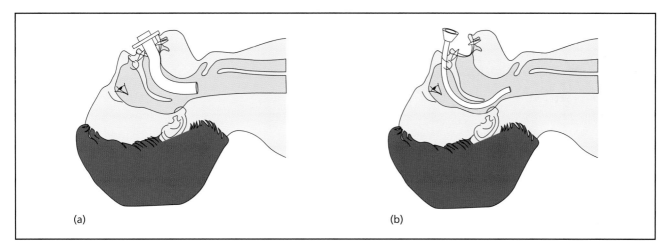

(a)   (b)

▲ **Fig. 54** Basic adjuncts to airway control: (**a**) oropharyngeal airway *in situ*; (**b**) nasopharyngeal airway *in situ*.

Insertion of a nasopharyngeal airway

Select an airway with an external diameter similar to the patient's little finger. Place a safety pin through the external flange of the airway to prevent it being inhaled. Lubricate the airway. Check the patency of the patient's nostrils and for the presence of septal deviation: use the nostril that seems easiest. Insert the airway perpendicularly to the nostril, along the floor of the nose. The airway should pass easily, such that the flange comes to rest at the nostril; if it does not, remove it and try the other nostril. Reassess the airway.

⚠ Do not insert a nasopharyngeal airway if there is a suspected fracture of the base of the skull.

Ventilatory support
Ventilatory support must be provided if the patient has inadequate or absent ventilation. In the short term, this can be provided by mouth-to-mouth, mouth-to-mask or bag-valve-mask ventilation (the latter is a two-person technique unless you are experienced). It is more important to ventilate the patient than for the inexperienced to attempt intubation. Get help!

3.7.2 Tracheostomy

Indications
There are two main indications for placement of a tracheostomy.

- Protection of the airway: following surgery to the head or neck; trauma or obstruction to the upper airway, eg smoke inhalation or facial burns; and bulbar or pseudobulbar palsies, to prevent aspiration and facilitate the clearance of secretions.

- Reduction in work of breathing (a tracheostomy reduces the dead space of the upper airways by about 150 mL or 50%): when weaning from ventilation, and in patients with chronic obstructive pulmonary disease or neuromuscular disorders.

Types of tracheostomy

Percutaneous tracheostomy
A cuffed tube is inserted (usually in the intensive care unit) following a blunt dissection of the tissues and serial dilation. A track becomes established about 10 days after placement, at which point the temporary tracheostomy should be changed to one with a removable inner tube to facilitate cleaning.

If a percutaneous tracheostomy becomes displaced within the first 7–10 days, before a track forms, then the tissues tend to spring back and prevent its safe replacement. Do not attempt to replace it: the patient should be re-intubated.

Formal tracheostomy
A cuffed tube, usually with a removable inner tube, is inserted by means of a surgical operation (typically in theatre), such that a track is formed immediately. If the tracheostomy becomes displaced it is often possible to open the track and replace it.

All patients with a formal tracheostomy should have a tracheostomy set including tracheostomy forceps at the bedside.

Mini-tracheostomy
This is an uncuffed tube used primarily to facilitate suctioning in patients with poor cough that may be placed in intensive care settings or occasionally on the ward.

Complications of tracheostomies
Immediate complications include haemorrhage, direct injury to the trachea or paratracheal structures, air embolism, apnoea and cardiac arrest. Early complications are:

- subcutaneous emphysema, pneumothorax or pneumomediastinum;

- tube displacement;

- tube blockage;

- infection;

- tracheal necrosis;

- difficulty swallowing.

Late complications include:

- haemorrhage;

- granuloma formation;

- tracheo-cutaneous or tracheo-oesophageal fistula;

- tracheal stenosis;

- scarring.

Principles of tracheostomy management

- Cleaning: the biggest concern with tracheostomies is obstruction, so it is essential that tracheostomies are kept clean; removable inner tubes should be inspected and cleaned regularly.

- Infection: the tracheostomy site should be inspected regularly and kept dry. Any moisture under the dressings will encourage skin breakdown, and infection at the site may compromise the airway.

- Humidification: inadequate humidification of inspired gas results in heat loss, moisture loss and hypoxia (functional residual capacity and static compliance fall due to atelectasis); excessive humidification can result in impairment of mucociliary clearance and surfactant activity.

- Suctioning: this will stimulate the cough reflex and prevent accumulation of secretions that can cause tracheostomy blockage. Suctioning systems may be open or closed, with the latter commonly used in the intensive care setting to reduce the risk of infection.

- Check cuff pressure: the inflation pressure of the cuff should be kept to a minimum to prevent trauma to the trachea, the recommended limit being 15–25 cmH$_2$O.

Changing a tracheostomy

Percutaneous temporary tracheostomies are generally changed at around 10 days when a track has formed. Formal tracheostomies may be changed for a different size or type depending on clinical circumstances. To change a tracheostomy, follow the procedure below.

- Full resuscitation facilities should be available in case of difficulties. Patients should be starved in case emergency reintubation is required and intravenous access should be available.

- The procedure should be explained to the patient: it is mildly unpleasant and often results in coughing.

- Organise monitoring: oxygen saturation and ECG.

- Remove any oropharyngeal secretions by suction.

- Deflate the cuff of the existing tracheostomy tube and remove it.

- Insert the new tracheostomy with inner tube into the track and inflate the cuff.

- Secure the new tracheostomy tube in place.

3.8 Ventilatory support

Respiratory failure may be divided in to type 1 (inadequate oxygenation) and type 2 (inadequate ventilation). Type 1 respiratory failure can be partially or completely treated with controlled oxygen therapy or continuous positive airway pressure (CPAP), and type 2 respiratory failure with non-invasive positive-pressure ventilation (NIPPV) or invasive positive-

pressure ventilation. Arterial blood gases (ABGs) should be obtained in all patients who are thought to have respiratory failure to determine its type and to guide management.

3.8.1 Controlled oxygen therapy

- Mild hypoxaemia (Pa_{O_2} >8.0 kPa): nasal prongs at 2–4 L/min or a Venturi mask at 24%.

- Moderate to severe hypoxaemia (Pa_{O_2} 6.7–8.0 kPa) without CO_2 retention: simple mask with 4–15 L/min depending on ABGs.

- Moderate hypoxaemia with CO_2 retention: use controlled oxygen therapy using a Venturi mask. Start at 24% oxygen and reassess ABGs at 20 minutes. If Pa_{O_2} <10 kPa and if Pa_{CO_2} has risen less than 1.3 kPa, increase oxygen to 28%. Recheck ABGs. If hypoxia persists with no deterioration in CO_2, consider further incremental increases in FI_{O_2} with close monitoring (ABGs). If hypercapnia progresses, NIPPV or invasive positive-pressure ventilation should be considered.

- Severe hypoxaemia (Pa_{O_2} <6.7 kPa): give high-flow oxygen via a reservoir mask and get immediate help.

Hypoxia kills quicker than hypercapnia

- All severely ill patients should receive high-flow oxygen.
- Patients with chronic obstructive pulmonary disease (COPD) who rely on their hypoxic drive for ventilation should receive high-flow oxygen initially if they are very ill. This may buy time to institute other therapies. If they improve, slowly reduce the FI_{O_2}; if they do not, consider ventilatory support.

3.8.2 Continuous positive airway pressure

CPAP is used in patients with acute type 1 respiratory failure when hypoxia persists despite high-flow oxygen supplementation. It enables a higher inspired oxygen concentration, reduces the work of breathing, improves lung compliance and recruits collapsed alveoli.

Indications

Acute pulmonary oedema, pneumonia and obstructive sleep apnoea.

Contraindications

- Haemodynamic instability.

- Life-threatening hypoxia.

- Exhaustion, impaired mental state, depressed conscious level (GCS <8) or confusion.

- Recent facial or upper airway surgery or facial pathology (eg burns).

- Recent upper gastrointestinal surgery.

- Inability to protect the airway; and copious secretions or vomitus.

A chest drain needs to be inserted prior to commencing CPAP in patients with a pneumothorax.

Practical considerations

CPAP is administered via a tight-fitting nasal or facial mask. The usual range of pressure supplied is 2.5–10 cmH$_2$O in conjunction with high-flow oxygen therapy. Alterations in settings are guided by oxygen saturations, blood gas analysis and the clinical situation. A wide-bore nasogastric tube should be inserted to enable decompression of the stomach.

Complications

Intolerance of face mask, air leaks, gastric distension, vomiting and aspiration, eye irritation and conjunctivitis, and facial skin necrosis.

3.8.3 Non-invasive ventilation

Non-invasive ventilation refers to the use of ventilatory support via a mask or similar device. It is vital that the ceiling of treatment is decided on in the event of treatment failure before commencing non-invasive ventilation: would invasive ventilation be considered? Bi-level positive airway pressure (BiPAP) is used in patients with type 2 (hypercapnic) respiratory failure.

Indications

BiPAP should be considered in patients with acute exacerbation of COPD who have respiratory acidosis (pH <7.35) despite maximal treatment; acute or acute-on-chronic hypercapnic respiratory failure is also an indication.

Contraindications

- Haemodynamic instability.

- Life-threatening hypoxia.

- Exhaustion, impaired mental state, depressed conscious level (GCS <8) or confusion.

- Recent facial or upper airway surgery or facial pathology (eg burns).

- Recent upper gastrointestinal surgery.

- Inability to protect the airway.

- Copious secretions or vomitus.

A chest drain needs to be inserted prior to commencing BiPAP in patients with a pneumothorax.

Practical considerations

BiPAP is administered via a tight-fitting nasal or facial mask. Typical initial settings in a patient with acute hypercapnic ventilatory failure are that the mode can be either spontaneous or timed and that expiratory positive airway pressure (EPAP) is 4–6 cmH$_2$O, inspiratory positive airway pressure 12–15 cmH$_2$O and back-up breaths 12–15/minute. It is important that patients are closely monitored for signs of both improvement and deterioration: ABGs should be measured 1 hour after commencing treatment or after setting changes. If there appears to be clinical decline or no objective evidence of clinical improvement after 4–6 hours, then invasive ventilation should be considered if appropriate.

Complications

- Intolerance of face mask, air leaks and ventilator–patient asynchrony.

- Gastric distension, vomiting and aspiration.

- Eye irritation and conjunctivitis.

- Facial skin necrosis.

3.8.4 Invasive ventilation

Invasive ventilation is applied via an endotracheal tube or tracheostomy. Ventilation is adjusted by altering the minute volume (respiratory rate × tidal volume). Oxygenation is adjusted by altering inspired oxygen concentration and positive end-expiratory pressure, which acts in a similar manner to CPAP/EPAP by recruiting collapsed alveoli and reducing the work of breathing.

Indications

- Airway protection, eg facial trauma or burns, and the unconscious patient.

- Reversible respiratory failure.

- Prophylactic ventilation, eg after major surgery where some degree of respiratory failure might be expected.

- To avoid or control hypercapnia, eg in acute head injury or hepatic coma.

- In 'flail' chest to act as an internal splint.

- To facilitate the removal of secretions, eg in Guillain–Barré syndrome and myasthenia gravis.

Practical considerations

Arrange the settings on the ventilator as follows for an adult: tidal volume 6–10 mL/kg, respiratory rate 10–14/minute and ratio of inspiratory to expiratory time (I:E ratio) <1. For patients with COPD or asthma the I:E ratio often needs to be smaller (eg 1:3) to prevent gas trapping and hyperinflation.

Control of the airway

The advantages of nasotracheal intubation compared with an endotracheal tube are that it is better tolerated by the conscious patient and fixation is more secure. Its disadvantages include damage to the nasal mucosa, alar cartilages and nasal septum; bronchial suction is more difficult; and it causes increased resistance to gas flow and an increased incidence of sinus infection.

Tracheostomy has the advantage over intubation of being better tolerated by patients, such that sedation can be reduced and weaning is often facilitated. Indications include prolonged ventilation, expected prolonged absence of protective laryngeal reflexes, retention of secretions, head and neck injuries/surgery, and upper airway obstruction. Complications include displacement of the tube, bleeding and infection; tracheal stenosis; and failure of the tracheostomy track to heal.

Types of ventilator

- Pressure generators: these produce a preset airway pressure or cycle from inspiration to expiration when a preset pressure is reached. If lung compliance falls or airway resistance increases, the tidal volume delivered will fall. This is the most commonly used mode in the intensive care setting.

- Volume generators: deliver a fixed tidal volume regardless of changes in lung mechanics. If the lungs become stiffer, the inflation pressure will increase to deliver the same tidal volume.

- Cycling: the change from inspiration to expiration is usually time cycled, but from expiration to inspiration it is either time cycled or triggered by the patient if breathing spontaneously.

General management of the ventilated patient

It is essential that the patient's breathing is synchronised to that of the ventilator. Failure to do so results in increased oxygen requirement, increased CO_2 production, reduced cardiac output and distress to the patient. Sedation by parenteral infusion of narcotics and short-acting benzodiazepines is generally used.

Inhaled gases should be warmed, humidified and filtered. Secretions should be cleared by regular physiotherapy and endotracheal suction. Pulse oximetry and measurement of end-tidal CO_2 provides continuous assessment of oxygenation and ventilation, and ABGs should be checked regularly.

Complications of invasive ventilation

- Ventilator-associated pneumonia: ventilated patients have a 10–20 times increased risk of acquiring pneumonia compared with non-ventilated patients.

- Lung damage: over-distension of the alveoli and other mechanical effects may exacerbate lung injury. High inflation pressures can cause pneumothorax or subcutaneous emphysema.

- Adverse haemodynamic effects: a raised intrathoracic pressure reduces venous return and increases pulmonary vascular resistance; furthermore, cardiac output and arterial blood pressure are reduced, and heart rate and systemic vascular resistance rise.

4.1 Self-assessment questions

Question 1

Clinical scenario

A 67-year-old man presents to the Emergency Department following a collapse at work. He has never collapsed before. His medical history includes hypertension, non-insulin-dependent diabetes mellitus and ischaemic heart disease. On examination his pulse is 40 bpm and his BP 80/40 mmHg. His ECG is shown in Fig. 55.

Question

What is the diagnosis?

Answers

A First-degree atrioventricular (AV) block
B Sinus bradycardia
C Second-degree AV block
D Third-degree AV block
E Sick sinus syndrome

Question 2

Clinical scenario

A 42-year-old man presents to the Emergency Department with a history of breathlessness and right-sided pleuritic chest pain of 48 hours' duration. He is normally fit and well, and takes no regular medication, but does admit to smoking 20–30 cigarettes/day. On examination his respiratory rate is 22/minute, his Sao_2 94% on air and his pulse 90 bpm, and in the chest he has reduced expansion and quiet breath sounds in the right hemithorax. Routine blood investigations are unremarkable, and his CXR is shown in Fig. 56.

Question

How would you manage this patient initially?

Answers

A Observation only is required; he could safely be discharged with follow-up in 7–10 days
B Aspiration with observation for 24 hours; CXR prior to discharge to check resolution; follow-up arranged for 4 weeks; and advice on smoking cessation

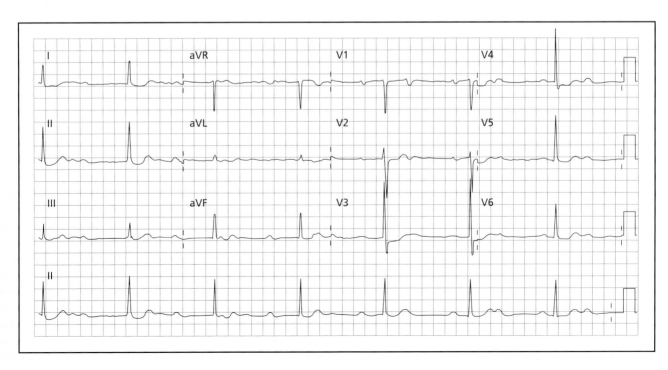

▲ **Fig. 55** Question 1.

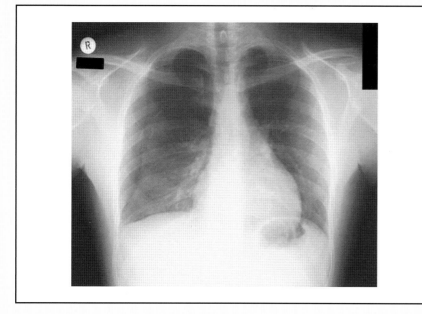

Fig. 56 Question 2.

C Admit; treat with oral amoxicillin

D Admit; treat with intravenous Augmentin (co-amoxiclav) and clarithromycin

E Admit; treat with intravenous cefotaxime

Question 4

Clinical scenario

A 19-year-old diabetic man is admitted with a 3-day history of nausea and vomiting. On examination he is apyrexial (36.5°C) with respiratory rate 28/minute, pulse 110 bpm and BP 100/65 mmHg. His abdomen is soft and non-tender and his chest is clear. Investigations reveal a fingerprick blood glucose of 28 mmol/L. Urine dipstick records protein + and ketones ++. Laboratory tests show C-reactive protein 12 mg/dL (normal <6), white cell count 14.3×10^9/L (normal range 4–11), potassium 3.1 mmol/L (normal range 3.5–5.0), urea 14.2 mmol/L (normal range 3–7), creatinine 123 μmol/L (normal range 60–115) and glucose 25.6 mmol/L (normal range 3–6.5). Arterial blood gases show pH 7.23

C Aspiration and discharge home after a CXR prior to discharge to check resolution; follow-up arranged for 4 weeks; and advice on smoking cessation

D Admission and insertion of 28Fr intercostal chest drain

E Admission and insertion of 12Fr intercostal chest drain

Question 3

Clinical scenario

A 72-year-old man is admitted from a residential home with a 3-day history of progressive confusion. Examination reveals he has pyrexia of 38.5°C, respiratory rate >30/minute, Sao_2 90% on air, pulse 120 bpm, BP 100/75 mmHg and in the chest there is a dull percussion note and bronchial breathing in the right upper zone. Investigations show C-reactive protein 253 mg/dL (normal <6), urea 10.2 mmol/L (normal range 3–7), creatinine 145 μmol/L (normal range 60–115) and white cell count 17.2×10^9/L (normal range 4–11). Figure 57 shows his CXR.

Question

How would you manage this man's illness?

Answers

A Discharge with oral amoxicillin and clarithromycin; arrange follow-up in 6–8 weeks

B Discharge with oral ciprofloxacin; arrange follow-up in 6–8 weeks

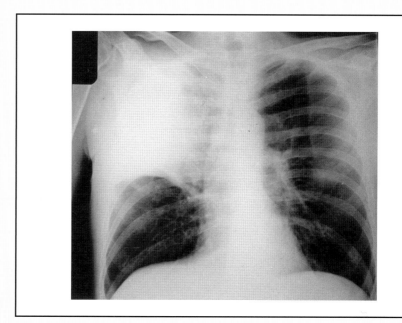

Fig. 57 Question 3.

and HCO$_3^-$ 12 mmol/L. The CXR is unremarkable.

Question
What is your initial management plan?

Answers
A Insulin infusion
B Fluid replacement with 0.9% saline
C Fluid replacement with 5% dextrose
D Fluid replacement with 0.9% saline (with K$^+$ supplementation), and also insulin infusion
E Fluid replacement with 5% dextrose (with K$^+$ supplementation), and also insulin infusion

Question 5

Clinical scenario
A 28-year-old woman with known asthma presents with an exacerbation. She cannot speak in sentences, has a respiratory rate of 32/minute and a pulse rate of 120 bpm. Her peak expiratory flow rate (PEFR) is 45% of predicted. Routine blood tests are normal, excepting an elevated white cell count (WCC) of 22 × 10^9/L (normal range 4–11).

Question
Which of these is *not* a feature of acute severe asthma?

Answers
A PEFR 45% predicted
B Respiratory rate 32/minute
C WCC 22 × 10^9/L
D Pulse rate 120 bpm
E Inability to complete a sentence

Question 6

Clinical scenario
A 32-year-old woman with a history of thyrotoxicosis caused by Graves' disease, who is taking carbimazole 20 mg three times daily and thyroxine 100 µg once daily as a

'block and replace' regimen, becomes generally weak and unwell. She is sent to the Emergency Department for assessment.

Question
Which of the following would you *not* expect to be a feature if she was presenting in addisonian crisis?

Answers
A BP 90/60 mmHg
B Serum potassium 3.1 mmol/L
C Blood glucose 4.0 mmol/L
D Vitiligo
E Serum sodium 128 mmol/L

Question 7

Clinical scenario
A 48-year-old man presents with a 3-week history of worsening breathlessness that has become much worse over the last 24 hours. He is finding it very difficult to speak or to swallow, is drooling saliva and has inspiratory stridor. Examination of his neck reveals bilateral palpable masses probably due to lymphadenopathy.

Question
Which of the following would *not* be appropriate in his initial management?

Answers
A High-flow oxygen therapy
B CT scan of the thorax/neck
C Intravenous high dose steroids
D Intubation and ventilation
E Intramuscular epinephrine (1 in 1,000, 0.5 mL)

Question 8

Clinical scenario
A 67-year-old man with a long history of alcohol abuse presents with abdominal pain. He has never had such a problem before. He looks unwell and has cool hands, pulse 110 bpm, BP 110/70 mmHg and tenderness with guarding across his

upper abdomen. On clinical grounds it is difficult to decide whether he has acute pancreatitis or peritonitis.

Question
Which of the following statements is true?

Answers
A Alcohol abuse causes chronic pancreatitis but not acute pancreatitis
B Discomfort in the lumbar region of the back is more likely in acute pancreatitis than in peritonitis
C A first presentation with acute pancreatitis is unlikely at the age of 67 years
D The diagnosis is unlikely to be acute pancreatitis if no pancreatic calcification is seen on an abdominal radiograph
E Serum amylase is a prognostic indicator in acute pancreatitis

Question 9

Clinical scenario
You are asked to review a 69-year-old woman in the Medical Assessment Unit. She is poorly responsive, with a Glasgow Coma Scale score of 9. The physician's assistant has already performed a 12-lead ECG (Fig. 58).

Question
What is the most likely underlying cause of this presentation?

Answers
A Hypothyroidism
B Myocardial infarction
C Hypothermia
D Beta-blocker overdose
E Hypoglycaemia

Question 10

Clinical scenario
A dishevelled man of about 30 years is brought to the resuscitation room of the Emergency Department by blue-light ambulance after being

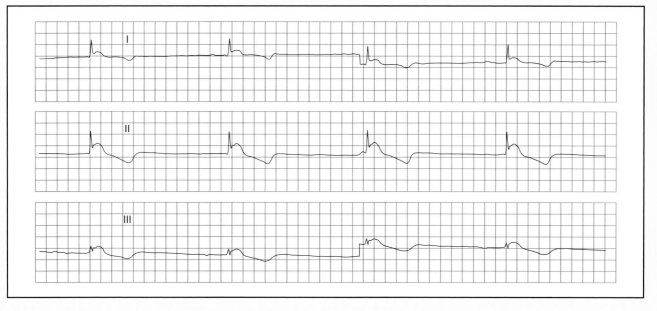

▲ **Fig. 58** Question 9.

found collapsed in the street. He is unable to speak and despite making substantial respiratory efforts he looks deeply cyanosed. His pulse is difficult to feel and you cannot record a BP. His chest looks asymmetrical, more prominent on the right side. On auscultation you cannot hear breath sounds over the right side of the chest, but you can hear a few in the left axilla. The heart sounds are difficult to hear and you cannot palpate the apex beat. You should:

Answers

A Get an urgent ECG

B Get an urgent CXR

C Get an urgent check of fingerprick blood glucose

D Urgently prepare for cardioversion

E Insert a needle into the right side of his chest

Question 11

Clinical scenario

A 22-year-old woman presents with a headache and a temperature. Yesterday she flew home from a

week's trip to a game reserve near Johannesburg, South Africa.

Question

Which one of the following statements is true?

Answers

A *Plasmodium falciparum* is unlikely if the fever started on day 5 of the trip

B Patients with malaria often have cervical lymphadenopathy

C Patients with malaria often have a maculopapular rash, particularly on the trunk

D Malaria has been eradicated from South Africa

E The presence of neutropenia would help to differentiate between typhoid and malaria

Question 12

Clinical scenario

A 50-year-old man with known inflammatory bowel disease is referred by his GP with a 3-day history of bloody diarrhoea. His wife has also been passing blood in her stool.

Question

Which one of the following is true?

Answers

A Appearance at sigmoidoscopy may not help differentiate between an infective colitis and an acute episode of inflammatory bowel disease

B The surgical team should be involved when the colon appears dilated >10 cm on a plain abdominal film

C Outbreaks of amoebiasis are rare in the UK

D There is no role for systemic steroids when an infective cause is the most likely reason for his symptoms

E His haemoglobin on admission is 10.5 g/dL: he should not be prescribed a prophylactic dose of low-molecular-weight heparin while an inpatient

Question 13

Clinical scenario

A 52-year-old woman presents with pleuritic chest pain and breathlessness. She appears anxious, but a physical examination is normal. The obvious concern is that she has suffered a pulmonary embolism (PE).

Question

Which one of the following statements is *not* true?

Answers

A An ischaemic ECG makes the diagnosis of PE less likely in a patient presenting with pleuritic chest pain

B Investigations for occult cancer are only indicated in PE when cancer is suspected clinically, on CXR or on routine blood tests

C D-dimer assay should not be performed in those with a high clinical probability of PE

D Thrombolysis is first-line treatment for massive PE and current British Thoracic Society guidelines recommend alteplase

E Unfractionated heparin should be considered as a first-dose bolus in massive PE or where rapid reversal of effect may be needed; otherwise low-molecular-weight heparin is preferable to unfractionated heparin

Question 14

Clinical scenario

An 18-year-old woman presents after taking an aspirin overdose. She is tearful and distressed but not suicidal and regrets having taken the tablets. She has tinnitus and is hyperventilating.

Question

Which one of the following statements is true?

Answers

A Activated charcoal should be given if she presents 8 hours after taking the overdose

B Gastric lavage is indicated if she presents 2 hours after taking the overdose

C Intravenous sodium bicarbonate is given to alkalinise the urine and enhance urinary salicylate excretion when the plasma salicylate concentration is greater than 700 mg/L (5.1 mmol/L) in adults

D Any patient who has tinnitus following an aspirin overdose should be referred for renal dialysis

E In aspirin overdose blood gases may show a respiratory alkalosis with a metabolic acidosis and a raised anion gap

Question 15

Clinical scenario

A 23-year-old woman is brought in at 10 o'clock one evening by her friends having taken an overdose of around 36 500-mg paracetamol tablets over the course of the day with a large amount of alcohol. They say that she is otherwise well, although they think she may have been anorexic in the past. At the moment she is vomiting and refusing all medical treatment.

Question

Which two of the following statements are *not* correct?

Answers

A You assume she has a mental illness and assess that her capacity is in doubt: your duty of care to her then allows you to treat her against her will and ultimately potentially save her life

B The history of anorexia puts her on the high-risk treatment line

C Liver damage is maximal 3–4 days after ingestion and may lead to encephalopathy, haemorrhage, hypoglycaemia, cerebral oedema and death

D She should not be prescribed activated charcoal

E In this situation the plasma paracetamol concentration

cannot be interpreted on the graph and because the total dose in 24 hours exceeds 150 mg/kg, *N*-acetylcysteine should be given

F Blood levels should be taken at 4 hours after the time the last tablets were taken and if the levels are above the high-risk treatment line, *N*-acetylcysteine should be given

G She needs a psychiatric assessment of her capacity prior to any treatment being instituted for the management of the overdose

H Oral methionine is ineffective if given any later than 12 hours from the overdose

I Patients who are known to be repeat overdose attenders are not included as a high-risk group if they have previously been fully treated with an antidote, as their glutathione stores will be replenished

J Start *N*-acetylcysteine immediately if patients present over 24 hours after the overdose and are symptomatic. If they are asymptomatic, check the patient for biochemical evidence of liver/renal damage before starting any antidote

Question 16

Clinical scenario

A 45-year-old man presents to the Emergency Department with back pain which came on after a day when he lifted a lot of heavy planks of wood off a lorry. He is a carpenter and has had some back pain over the years, but nothing like this. Paracetamol has not helped. He has no other symptoms and an examination is normal, except that the left ankle jerk is difficult to elicit.

Question

Which of the following statements is *not* true?

Answers

A When discharging patients with non-specific low back pain they should be advised to avoid bed-rest and stay active

B Over 90% of patients with non-specific low back pain will recover within 6 weeks

C The presence of a unilateral absent ankle jerk suggests the need for an urgent MRI scan

D In the management of non-specific low back pain muscle relaxants will have no effect on the outcome, although they may improve symptoms

E Any patient with difficulty urinating requires urgent further investigation

Question 17

Clinical scenario

A 40-year-old man is brought to the Emergency Department by the police on a section. They were involved when he was witnessed in the street as behaving in an extremely disturbed way. He has a large laceration at the occiput. He is currently behaving in an aggressive manner towards other patients and staff. You are called to assess.

Question

Which one of the following statements is *not* true?

Answers

A The police will have employed section 136 to bring the patient to a place of safety

B You should consider sedating this patient if de-escalation techniques fail

C In order to exclude a significant head injury the Mental Health Act should be applied to allow assessment and treatment

D As a registered medical practitioner you are able to assess a patient's capacity

E Intravenous haloperidol should not be used for emergency sedation

Question 18

Clinical scenario

A 62-year-old man has been referred from the Emergency Department with an acute coronary syndrome. He has dynamic ST-segment changes but is currently pain-free. He is receiving maximal medical treatment when you are called to see him urgently because his BP has fallen to 80/50 mmHg.

Question

Which of the following statements is *not* true?

Answers

A Sudden recurrence of the chest pain and a fall in BP is suggestive of cardiac rupture

B If on examination he has a raised JVP and a clear chest, then a fluid bolus should be tried

C Rapid onset of hypotension and breathlessness is suggestive of left ventricular failure

D Inotropes should be used with caution because they will increase afterload through an increase in systemic vascular resistance and lead to further demands on myocardial oxygen consumption

E The first action you should take is to stop the intravenous nitrate

Question 19

Clinical scenario

A 68-year-old man presents with chest pain. On the basis of history, examination and ECG a diagnosis of non-ST-elevation myocardial infarction is made.

Question

Which one of the following is *not* one of the seven risk factors for the calculation of the Thrombolysis in Myocardial Infarction risk score?

Answers

A Aspirin use within the last 7 days

B T-wave inversion in leads other than III, aVR or V1

C Coronary artery stenosis greater than 50%

D Age over 65 years

E Raised cardiac markers

Question 20

Clinical scenario

A 72-year-old woman with no significant past medical history apart from hypertension, for which she takes bendroflumethiazide 2.5 mg once daily, presents with breathlessness that has developed over the last 24 hours. She is aware that her pulse 'went funny' at about the time the problem started. On examination she is in atrial fibrillation (AF) at a rate of 150/minute and has bibasal crackles.

Question

In managing someone who presents with new-onset AF, which of the following is true?

Answers

A The patient should receive heparin in the absence of contraindications

B If the patient has had AF for >48 hours or the duration of AF is uncertain, start anticoagulant treatment before an attempt is made to restore sinus rhythm

C If the patient has had AF for >48 hours or the duration of AF is uncertain, then antithrombotic treatment should be followed by rhythm control with intravenous amiodarone

D A haemodynamically stable patient with chest pain, fast AF and left ventricular dysfunction should be given intravenous verapamil to control the rate

E Digoxin should be used for rate limitation if the patient with fast AF has ventricular pre-excitation

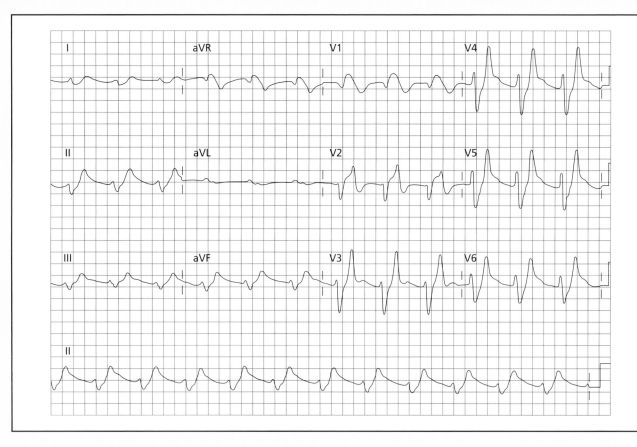

▲ **Fig. 59** Question 22.

Question 21

Clinical scenario

A 53-year-old woman is found collapsed at home with a Glasgow Coma Scale score of 4 (E1, V1, M2). She has a fixed and dilated right pupil.

Question

Which of the following is the most likely diagnosis?

Answers

A Hypoglycaemia
B Opioid overdose
C Total anterior circulation syndrome
D Acute extradural haemorrhage
E Acute subarachnoid haemorrhage

Question 22

Clinical scenario

A 63-year-old man has become progressively more short of breath following bilateral hip replacements.

He denies a history of chest pain. His ECG is shown in Fig. 59.

Question

Which of the following is the most likely diagnosis?

Answers

A Ventricular tachycardia
B Hyperkalaemia
C Pulmonary embolism
D Acute anterior myocardial infarction
E Supraventricular tachycardia with right bundle branch block

Question 23

Clinical scenario

A man who appears to be about 20 years old is brought to the Emergency Department having been found unconscious in the street. His airway, breathing and circulation are satisfactory. His fingerprick blood glucose is 4.2 mmol/L.

Question

You proceed to check his Glasgow Coma Scale (GCS) score: which of the following are required to do this?

Answers

A Pupillary size, best motor response and best verbal response
B Best verbal response, best motor response and best eye opening response
C Best verbal response, lateralising signs and pupillary size
D Localising signs, best eye opening response and best verbal response
E Pupillary size, best verbal response and lateralising signs

Question 24

Clinical scenario

A 35-year-old man attends the Emergency Department with a 36-hour history of progressive swelling of his left hand following a dog bite. On examination there is cellulitis and a small puncture wound exuding pus on the thenar eminence. He also has some tender axillary lymphadenopathy. He has no drug allergies.

Question

What is the most appropriate antibiotic treatment?

Answers

A Erythromycin
B Benzylpenicillin and flucloxacillin
C Doxycycline
D Ceftriaxone
E Co-amoxiclav

Question 25

Clinical scenario

A 28-year-old nursing assistant with a history of anxiety and depression presents to the Emergency Department with acute dyspnoea. She also complains of parathesiae affecting both hands.

Question

Which set of blood gas results (with the patient breathing air) is consistent with hyperventilation?

Answers

	pH	Pa_{O_2} (kPa)	Pa_{CO_2} (kPa)	Bicarbonate (mmol/L)
Normal	7.36–7.44	11.3–13.0	4.5–6.0	19–24
A	6.90	12.9	3.0	10
B	7.50	7.9	4.0	20
C	7.52	12.5	3.5	19
D	7.28	12.8	2.8	12
E	7.32	7.0	8.2	34

Question 26

Clinical scenario

A 36-year-old man presents in a confused state. He has Down's syndrome and his care worker has witnessed him having two generalised tonic–clonic seizures. She tells you that he had just started a course of antibiotics for an ear

infection and that he had a 'skin cancer' removed several years ago, but has no other past history. On examination, his temperature is 37.5°C, he is drowsy, and he has a stiff neck and a purulent discharge from his right ear. His BP is 200/120 mmHg. He has bilateral papilloedema. Both plantar responses are extensor. He undergoes an urgent CT scan of the head (non-contrast). This shows several areas of low attenuation involving both cerebral hemispheres. Evidence of haemorrhage is present in several of these areas.

Question

What is the most likely diagnosis?

Answers

A Metastatic malignant melanoma
B Hypertensive encephalopathy
C Subarachnoid haemorrhage
D Primary intracerebral haemorrhage
E Cortical thrombophlebitis

Question 27

Clinical scenario

A 40-year-old man who has a known prawn allergy developed an urticarial rash 3 hours after eating

a meal thought to contain a small amount of shellfish. He has a history of asthma. On examination 1 hour after his rash began he was anxious with a pulse rate of 100 bpm, BP 150/100 mmHg and a respiratory rate of 30/minute. Pulse oximetry (on air) shows oxygen saturation 99%.

Question

What would be the most appropriate next step in management?

Answers

A Close observation
B Intramuscular epinephrine
C Subcutaneous epinephrine
D Intravenous epinephrine
E Discharge home

Question 28

Clinical scenario

A 40-year-old woman presents 4 hours after an overdose of diazepam and amitriptyline. On examination her Glasgow Coma Scale (GCS) score is 10, she has bilateral dilated pupils and a pulse rate of 140 bpm with BP 108/64 mmHg. Pulse oximetry (on air) shows oxygen saturation 95%.

Question

What is the most appropriate immediate management?

Answers

A Administration of activated charcoal
B Administration of intravenous atenolol
C Administration of intravenous flumazenil
D Check ECG
E CT scan of head

Question 29

Clinical scenario

A 50-year-old schoolteacher presents with a sudden-onset severe headache and vomiting. On examination he has meningism and a left oculomotor nerve palsy. A CT scan of his head reveals a subarachnoid haemorrhage.

Question

Which artery is the most likely site of the aneurysm?

Answers

A Anterior cerebral

B Anterior communicating

C Basilar

D Vertebral

E Posterior communicating

Question 30

Clinical scenario

A 18-year-old woman presents 7 hours after taking 24 g of paracetamol.

Question

Which factor is most likely to predict an increased risk of hepatotoxicity from paracetamol?

Answers

A Anorexia nervosa

B Consumption of two cans of 'extra strength' lager since taking the paracetamol

C Gilbert's disease

D Smoking 10 cigarettes per day

E A history of deliberate self-harm

Question 31

Clinical scenario

A 75-year-old man with hypertension presents with severe sudden-onset interscapular pain. On examination he has a grade 2 early diastolic murmur audible at the left sternal edge. His BP is 200/112 mmHg in his right arm and 162/92 mmHg in his left arm. An ECG shows left bundle branch block, CXR reveals a widened mediastinum and a transthoracic echocardiogram demonstrates moderate aortic regurgitation and a dilated aortic root.

Question

What is the most appropriate immediate drug therapy?

Answers

A Clopidogrel

B Ramipril

C Intravenous glyceryl trinitrate

D Intravenous labetalol

E Oral nifedipine

Question 32

Clinical scenario

A 50-year-old man is admitted with confusion and diarrhoea. On examination he has evidence of severe community-acquired pneumonia. Investigations reveal serum sodium 120 mmol/L (normal range 136–144), potassium 3.5 mmol/L (normal range 3.5–5.0), urea 12.0 mmol/L (normal range 2.5–7.2), white cell count 12×10^9/L (normal range 4–11) and the CXR shows bilateral consolidation.

Question

Which test is most useful in confirming the diagnosis of Legionnaires' disease?

Answers

A Induced sputum culture

B Serum indirect fluorescent antibody test

C Urinary antigen testing

D Bronchoalveolar lavage

E Direct immunofluorescent test on sputum

Question 33

Clinical scenario

A 50-year-old man who has consumed 10 units of alcohol per day for the last 15 years and has a 30 pack-year smoking history is admitted to hospital with unstable angina. He requires diamorphine and metoclopramide, and because of continuing nausea is commenced on a 5% dextrose infusion; 72 hours after admission he develops confusion and double vision.

Question

What is the most appropriate immediate drug treatment?

Answers

A Diazepam

B Haloperidol

C Lorazepam

D Thiamine

E Procyclidine

4.2 Self-assessment answers

Answer to Question 1

D

The ECG shows third-degree (complete) heart block, with P waves completely dissociated from the QRS complexes. The narrow QRS complexes indicate that the focus for ventricular activity is high in the ventricular conducting system. The patient has signs of circulatory collapse as a result of the bradycardia and it thus becomes imperative to act to obtain cardiac stability. The treatment of choice is temporary transvenous pacing, although atropine and isoprenaline may have a role to play.

Answer to Question 2

B

The history given and the results of the investigations are compatible with a primary pneumothorax. Although this man smokes there is no clear history of underlying comorbid lung disease, but this must be considered. He exhibits mild symptoms and is not overtly tachypnoeic or tachycardic. His CXR shows a large pneumothorax (visible rim of air >2 cm). The recommended treatment in this situation is aspiration, with observation if successful for 24 hours prior to discharge. If aspiration proves unsuccessful, the next step would be insertion of a small-bore (12–14Fr) chest drain. Smoking cessation advice is essential to reduce the risk of recurrence and should be offered to all patients who smoke. Follow-up arranged before discharge, in addition to general advice, is essential.

Answer to Question 3

D

The history, examination and investigation results are compatible with a diagnosis of right upper lobe pneumonia. According to the CURB-65 score he has severe pneumonia (confusion, urea >7 mmol/L, respiratory rate >30/minute and age >65; score 4/5) that necessitates hospital admission. Treatment with intravenous Augmentin (co-amoxiclav) in addition to a macrolide would be appropriate (British Thoracic Society guidelines 2004). A third-generation cephalosporin may be used as an alternative in conjunction with a macrolide.

Answer to Question 4

D

The diagnosis is diabetic ketoacidosis. The priority for management is fluid and electrolyte replacement. Patients are often severely dehydrated and very depleted of both sodium and potassium. The serum potassium concentration may be high at presentation, but will fall rapidly as it moves into cells with rehydration and insulin treatment.

Answer to Question 5

C

The features of acute severe asthma (British Thoracic Society guidelines 2003) include a peak expiratory flow rate of 33–50% predicted/best, an inability to complete a sentence in one breath, a respiratory rate >25/minute and a pulse rate >110 bpm.

Answer to Question 6

B

Acute addisonian crisis is classically associated with hypotension and tachycardia, and laboratory investigations showing hyponatraemia, hyperkalaemia and hypoglycaemia. A short Synacthen test would confirm the diagnosis. Areas of vitiligo are seen as an autoimmune association in Addison's disease.

Answer to Question 7

B

Initial management of the patient with stridor must be to stabilise the airway, if necessary by intubation. High-flow oxygen therapy and high-dose intravenous steroids should be given, and for patients *in extremis* intramuscular epinephrine (adrenaline) may need to be considered. A CT scan of the thorax/neck may be required following initial treatment and stabilisation of the airway, but putting this man into a scanner now is likely to be fatal.

Answer to Question 8

B

Acute and chronic pancreatitis may be seen in alcohol abuse. Pancreatic pain is typically felt in the epigastrium, but there is often a lot of associated discomfort in the lumbar region of the back. Pancreatitis is a potential cause of generalised abdominal pain and can mimic the peritonism of a ruptured viscus. Pancreatic calcification is present in chronic pancreatitis, but its absence does not exclude the diagnosis of acute pancreatitis. Serum amylase is a useful biochemical marker of acute pancreatitis, but is not an indicator of prognosis: the Ranson score

(prognostic scoring system) used in acute pancreatitis does not incorporate the serum amylase.

Answer to Question 9

C

The ECG shows sinus bradycardia, first-degree heart block and prominent 'J' waves, which are seen immediately after the QRS complex in hypothermia. These disappear with warming of the body temperature. The mechanism is not known.

Answer to Question 10

E

This man has a tension pneumothorax: urgent needle thoracocentesis should be performed and any of the other courses of action described could be fatal.

Answer to Question 11

A

Even if a malaria-infected mosquito had bitten her on the first day of her trip, the life cycle demands at least 7 days before the first symptoms appear, thus excluding malaria. Malaria does not cause rash or lymphadenopathy. Neutropenia may be found in both typhoid and malaria.

Answer to Question 12

A

The sigmoidoscopic appearance of infectious colitis and chronic idiopathic inflammatory bowel disease may be indistinguishable. The mucosal appearance of *Clostridium difficile* infection is also variable, although the adherent yellow-white plaques, or 'pseudomembrane', are characteristic. The surgical team should be involved early, particularly when there is a suspicion of superadded infection. Amoebiasis can be contracted in the UK. Treatment should include systemic steroids as well as antibiotics. The patient is at high risk for systemic thromboembolism and should be given prophylactic low-molecular-weight heparin.

Answer to Question 13

A

A pulmonary embolism (PE) may cause a sudden increase in the afterload on the right ventricle leading to ischaemia (in addition to hypoxia), which may precipitate left- or right-sided ischaemic changes on the ECG when there is underlying coronary artery disease. There is an increased risk of malignancy being detected within 6–12 months of a first episode of PE, particularly in those with no other risk factors and/or recurrent episodes. Occult cancer, present in 7–12% of those with apparently idiopathic PE, can usually be detected by a combination of careful clinical assessment, routine blood tests and CXR. This is true according to current British Thoracic Society guidelines, which also state that D-dimer alone is not a valid routine screening investigation for PE, and that it should only be used in conjunction with pretest clinical probability assessment.

If there has been a massive PE, ie one so severe as to cause circulatory collapse, the recommended practice is to use thrombolysis, the earlier the better, although evidence for a reduction in mortality is sparse. Low-molecular-weight heparin has equal efficacy and safety, and is easier to use.

Answer to Question 14

E

Activated charcoal is the preferred method of gut decontamination if the dose of toxin taken is significant: a single dose of charcoal (50 g for adults) can be given up to 2 hours after ingestion, and this can be extended to 6 hours for drugs that delay gastric emptying (which includes salicylates). Sodium bicarbonate (1.26%) is given to enhance urinary salicylate excretion when the plasma salicylate concentration is greater than 500 mg/L (3.6 mmol/L) in adults. Haemodialysis is the treatment of choice for severe salicylate poisoning and should be considered when the plasma salicylate concentration exceeds 700 mg/L (5.1 mmol/L) or in the presence of severe metabolic acidosis.

Answer to Question 15

F and G

Administration of activated charcoal should be considered if paracetamol in excess of 150 mg/kg or 12 g (whichever is the smaller) is thought to have been ingested within the previous hour. The plasma paracetamol concentration should be checked in all patients suspected of having taken an overdose: blood should be taken at 4 hours post ingestion. If the paracetamol level is not available within 8 hours of ingestion, then commence the antidotal therapy without awaiting the level. Stop treatment if the level is non-toxic. An accurate history is essential for the interpretation of the plasma paracetamol concentration; if there is any doubt then N-acetylcysteine should be given regardless of the levels. In the situation where the patient has taken the tablets over a period of time, in a staggered fashion (eg

more than 2 hours between doses) or where the time of ingestion is unknown, then the plasma paracetamol concentration cannot be interpreted on the graph and if the total dose in 24 hours exceeds 150 mg/kg or 12 g (whichever is the smaller; >75 mg/kg in high-risk patients), then N-acetylcysteine should be given.

It is reasonable to call on psychiatric services to make an assessment of capacity, but in this case there is insufficient time to do this. You must be able to assess capacity and then proceed with urgent treatment: this can be done in good faith, provided you are acting in her best interests and in line with a responsible body of medical opinion.

Answer to Question 16

C

Although back pain is a huge problem, the prognosis is good for most patients. Red flags from the history and on examination include significant injury; past medical history of cancer; first presentation <20 or >55 years; systemic upset (fever and weight loss); steroid treatment; intravenous drug use; thoracic pain; multilevel neurological signs or symptoms; structural deformity; pain that is constant, progressive and unrelenting; or difficulty with bladder or bowels.

Answer to Question 17

C

A section 136 is the police admission order that enables a police officer to remove a person apparently suffering from a mental disorder from a public place to a designated place of safety (usually the police station or the local Emergency Department) for assessment by a doctor and a social worker. A section

135 enables the police officer to enter the place of residence of a person they believe to be suffering from a mental disorder to take he or she to a place of safety.

The Mental Health Act does not apply to the detention and treatment of patients for physical illness, for which they must be either consenting or treated under the common law. Pre-registration doctors (Foundation Year 1) are not able to assess a patient's capacity. If the patient is judged as not having the capacity to refuse treatment, there is a clear duty of care towards the patient to assess and treat any possible head injury.

When de-escalation techniques fail and pharmacological methods have to be employed, the current recommendation is the use of a benzodiazepine for sedation with an antipsychotic. The newer atypical antipsychotics can be used in this situation (po or im). Haloperidol is still widely used, although it should only be given intramuscularly or orally: intravenous administration may cause life-threatening arrhythmias.

Answer to Question 18

C

Hypotension and breathlessness from left ventricular dysfunction will be of gradual onset. Right ventricular infarction is preload dependent and it is important that these patients receive fluid loading early. Inotropes should be seen as a holding mechanism pending revascularisation. Pharmacologically induced hypotension is common.

Answer to Question 19

B

The Thrombosis in Myocardial Infarction (TIMI) risk score is used to calculate risk in the management of patients with unstable angina/non-ST-elevation myocardial infarction acute coronary syndrome. It is based on the presence or absence of seven independent prognostic risk factors for early death and myocardial infarction. Those patients with a score >3 have been shown to benefit from early intervention. It is based on factors from the history, including the age of the patient (>65 years), the presence of at least three recognised risk factors for coronary artery disease, the finding at coronary angiography of a stenosis of greater than 50% and the use of aspirin within the last week. It also incorporates the current presentation including severe angina within the past 24 hours, raised cardiac markers and ST-segment change >0.5 mm.

Answer to Question 20

A

Anticoagulation should be initiated, but this must not delay any emergency intervention. If haemodynamically unstable with AF, then the patient's life is under threat and he or she should be cardioverted immediately irrespective of the duration of the AF. If the AF has been present for >48 hours the priority, after antithrombotic treatment, is rate control with intravenous beta-blockade or digoxin. In haemodynamically stable patients where the AF is of recent onset, the patient should undergo electrical cardioversion, and if that fails pharmacological cardioversion should be attempted. Amiodarone is both antiarrhythmic and rate limiting. Alternatives include digoxin, particularly in the presence of left ventricular dysfunction, and intravenous beta-blockade. Verapamil has a significant negatively inotropic effect and must be avoided where there is left ventricular dysfunction. If the patient is thought to be at low risk of recurrence of AF, then antithrombotic treatment should be discontinued. If the patient has ventricular pre-excitation (eg Wolff–Parkinson–White syndrome), then atrioventricular node-blocking drugs (including digoxin) should be avoided because they cause an increase in the pre-excitation and may precipitate ventricular fibrillation.

Answer to Question 21

E

All these diagnoses could cause coma, but the fixed and dilated right pupil makes the most likely diagnosis subarachnoid haemorrhage caused by a posterior communicating artery aneurysm (affecting the third nerve).

Answer to Question 22

B

The ECG shows features of severe hyperkalaemia, with flattened P waves, widened QRS complexes and tall peaked T waves. The patient has almost certainly gone into acute or acute-on-chronic renal failure postoperatively.

Answer to Question 23

B

The GCS comprises the best verbal response, the best motor response and the best eye opening response on a scale of 3–15. Pupillary size and reaction and the presence of lateralising signs are not part of the GCS but are important parts of the assessment of unconscious patients.

Answer to Question 24

E

Most infected dog-bite wounds yield polymicrobial organisms. *Pasteurella multocida* and *Staphylococcus aureus* are the most common aerobic organisms, occurring in 20–30% of infected dog-bite wounds. Other possible aerobic pathogens include *Streptococcus* species, *Corynebacterium* species, *Eikenella corrodens* and *Capnocytophaga canimorsus* (formerly known as DF-2). Anaerobic organisms, including *Bacteroides fragilis*, *Fusobacterium* species and *Veillonella parvula*, have also been implicated in infected dog bites.

Co-amoxiclav (Augmentin) is the antibiotic of choice for a dog bite. For patients who are allergic to penicillin, doxycycline (Vibramycin) is an acceptable alternative, except for children younger than 8 years and pregnant women. Where compliance is a concern, daily intramuscular ceftriaxone can be used. Erythromycin can be used in penicillin-allergic patients but has a higher failure rate.

Answer to Question 25

C

Only this answer is compatible with primary respiratory alkalosis. A and D show metabolic acidosis with secondary respiratory alkalosis; B shows hypoxia stimulating secondary respiratory alkalosis; and E shows type 2 respiratory failure, with a primary respiratory acidosis with secondary metabolic alkalosis.

Answer to Question 26

E

Thrombophlebitis can result in venous occlusion. Once the vein is occluded, the thrombus may extend to veins that drain into the sinus and result in cortical venous infarction with petechial or overtly haemorrhagic perivascular venous infarction. These commonly occur within the white matter or at the grey–white matter junction, and they do not conform to arterial distribution infarcts.

Answer to Question 27

A

He has no evidence of anaphylaxis and does not require epinephrine (adrenaline) at this stage. In view of his documented allergy and rash he will require observation and further drug treatment may be required (including antihistamines).

Answer to Question 28

D

The first priority, as always, is to ensure that airway, breathing and circulation are maintained. In this scenario we have no evidence of hypoxia or shock. If flumazenil were ineffective, further airway support may be required if the GCS were to decrease or hypoxia to develop. But in this scenario the ECG is the most appropriate immediate management as it is the most useful guide for indicating the potential for future arrhythmias: the wider the QRS complex, the higher the risk (>140 ms). Activated charcoal needs to be given soon after an overdose to be effective, and certainly within an hour: it should not be given to someone at risk of aspiration (decreased GCS).

Answer to Question 29

E

The oculomotor nerve (cranial nerve III) is anatomically close to the posterior communicating artery, so external compression of the oculomotor nerve can occur with aneurysms involving this artery.

Answer to Question 30

A

Cytochrome P450 2E1 (CYP2E1) converts paracetamol to a highly reactive intermediary metabolite, *N*-acetyl-*p*-benzoquinone imine (NAPQI). Chronic excessive alcohol consumption can induce CYP2E1, thus increasing the potential toxicity of paracetamol. Fasting is a risk factor, possibly because of depletion of hepatic glutathione reserves. Concomitant use of other drugs which induce cytochrome P450 enzymes, such as antiepileptics (including carbamazepine and phenytoin), have also been reported as risk factors.

Answer to Question 31

D

This man has an acute aortic dissection and will need urgent transfer to a cardiothoracic unit for urgent assessment once he has been stabilised. He must have strict BP control, the target being a mean arterial pressure of 60–75 mmHg. Labetalol is the drug of choice as it combines both α_1- and β-adrenergic blocking properties, and can be carefully titrated to reduce shear forces on the aorta. Intravenous glyceryl trinitrate will lower BP but may cause a reflex tachycardia.

Answer to Question 32

C

Legionella pneumophila is a Gram-negative rod but is not readily seen on Gram stain of sputum, where the presence of many leucocytes without any microorganisms visible raises the likelihood of an atypical pneumonia. The urinary antigen test for *Legionella* species is the most useful diagnostic test: it can be done rapidly and is sensitive and highly specific. However, the definitive method for diagnosis remains isolation of the organism from respiratory secretions (including sputum), but culture results typically take 3–5 days to become available.

Answer to Question 33

D

A man with a history of chronic alcohol excess presenting with diplopia and confusion has Wernicke's encephalopathy until proved otherwise. This is a medical emergency and should be treated with high-dose intravenous thiamine, usually given as a combination of B-group vitamins as an intravenous preparation (Pabrinex). The onset of Wernicke's encephalopathy may be acute, subacute or chronic. The classic triad of symptoms (confusion, ataxia and ophthalmoplegia) may be absent in many cases, and the diagnosis is easily missed because many acutely intoxicated patients are both confused and ataxic. Carbohydrate loading is a recognised precipitant; hence the 5% dextrose infusion may be of relevance in this case.

THE MEDICAL MASTERCLASS SERIES

Haematology and Oncology

HAEMATOLOGY

ONCOLOGY

Cardiology and Respiratory Medicine

CARDIOLOGY

RESPIRATORY MEDICINE

Gastroenterology and Hepatology

GASTROENTEROLOGY AND HEPATOLOGY

Neurology, Ophthalmology and Psychiatry

NEUROLOGY

PACES Stations and Acute Scenarios 3

Nephrology

NEPHROLOGY

Rheumatology and Clinical Immunology

RHEUMATOLOGY AND CLINICAL IMMUNOLOGY

INDEX

Note: page numbers in *italics* refer to figures, those in **bold** refer to tables.